When Health Care Hurts

When Health Care Hurts

Ten common assumptions that can
derail your care
&
How to get back on track

Elizabeth L. Bewley

AUTHOR'S NOTE

Nothing in this book should be interpreted as personal medical advice. Consult a qualified medical professional before you start, delay, change, or stop any treatment. Failure to consult a qualified medical professional could cause you serious harm or even death. The author and publisher expressly disclaim responsibility for any consequences of using the information in this book.

To protect privacy, names and identifying details have been changed unless the sources asked that I use their real names. All the stories are true except the one about Charles, in Chapter 8. His story is typical but does not describe the experience of one specific individual.

In places, *When Health Care Hurts* draws on my earlier book, *Killer Cure*. That said, 21 of the 25 patient stories based on first-hand interviews or personal experience are new. Some of the material expands on content that first appeared in my newspaper column, "The Good Patient," which appears weekly in the Prescott, AZ, *Daily Courier*.

For more information, please refer to www.elizabethbewley.net

COVER PHOTO

This train wreck in Maricopa County, AZ, was photographed in 1902 by an unknown photographer and is part of a Library of Congress collection. The term "train wreck" has become a metaphor for disasters, especially those that arise from incompatible viewpoints. People may see train wrecks coming but feel powerless to prevent them. *When Health Care Hurts* can help you both recognize impending train wrecks in health care and understand how to avoid them.

ISBN-10:1497546907
ISBN-13:978-1497546905

Do what you can, where you are, with what you have.

Theodore Roosevelt

Contents

Discussion

Additional Resources

Preface

I was an executive with health care icon Johnson & Johnson for 20 years. I arrived at J&J with an MBA from Columbia and later enrolled in additional master's level courses to learn more about how health care works. I was drawn to J&J because I had seen evidence that it put customers first. All my work rests on this one basic idea: that patients—the customers of health care—should come first.

When people seek help from the health care system, they embark on a journey that can be costly, time-consuming, difficult, and stressful. They do it anyway, expecting to be better off as a result. Often, the promise of health care is fulfilled and their lives are saved or dramatically improved.

Research shows, however, that health care also often goes awry, and people are harmed instead of helped. The first ten chapters of *When Health Care Hurts* highlight ten flawed assumptions that routinely drive the actions of doctors, nurses, and other health care professionals. These experts mean well, but often do not appreciate the damage that can result when they act on these mistaken beliefs.

The cumulative effect of these dangerous assumptions is that health care often does not put patients first. Instead, it behaves as if its purpose is *to deliver tests and treatments*. I propose a different purpose: *to enable people to lead the lives they want*.

I wrote *When Health Care Hurts* to help you get the great benefits health care offers while avoiding the harm it too often delivers.

The layout of the book makes it easy to focus on content that interests you:

- Thirty **true-life stories** (and one fictional one) are set off in italics, and vividly reveal the surprising ways in which care can fall apart.
- Thirty full-page **"How To" Action Guides** list easy-to-follow steps you can take to get what you need from health care and avoid harm.
- Nearly six dozen corner boxes offer **Sad But True** statistics showing that the stories reflect common problems.
- **Discussions** of research and lessons learned appear in regular type, expanding on both the stories and the statistics.
- Several **Figures** offer graphics to enhance the written material.
- The **Readers' Discussion Guide** offers almost a hundred questions that both summarize key points and offer a basis for discussion.
- Nearly three hundred **Notes** detail research sources and also offer additional quotations, analyses, and explanations.

Stories, action guides, statistics, and figures are all easy to find, as each has its own index, before the general index begins at the back of the book.

A note about terminology: I use the terms "health care" and "the health care system" as shorthand to avoid repeatedly listing all the players who have a role in diagnosing and treating people, including those who run hospitals and manufacture products used in treatment. I refer to "you" in comments that also apply to family members, friends, colleagues, and others you care about.

I wish you all the best as you pursue health care that *enables you to lead the life you want.*

"We have the best health care in the world"

Health care professionals in the U.S. are highly educated and well-intentioned. Medical research provides stunning advances that yield miracles. We spend more money on medical care per person than any other country does. At the same time, unintended errors in care are common, and even minor mistakes can result in devastating problems for patients.

Small errors, big consequences

Bob was born with four holes in his heart. One of them was larger than his aorta. Experts deemed it the most severe and complicated case they had ever seen. His doctors didn't tell his parents, Shannon and Jeff, that their baby was likely to die—but Bob deteriorated before their eyes.

He started turning blue when feeding and soon refused to eat at all; sucking was too much work for his weakened heart. A feeding tube was inserted, and night after night his parents set the alarm to wake up every three hours to feed him. Each feeding took an hour, and Bob vomited up most of what he took in.

His doctors wanted him to gain weight before he had surgery, which was almost certain to be futile anyway. But at three months, he weighed little more than he had at birth. He didn't look like a newborn, though. His head—which was normal-sized—looked huge in comparison to his tiny arms and legs. His body was channeling all the energy it could to his brain, to keep him alive.

SAD BUT TRUE

1 in 7

Patients age 65 or older who are seriously harmed or die because of mistakes in their care in the hospital

Inspector General of the United States Department of Health & Human Services in 2010, after studying a sample drawn from the nearly one million Medicare patients hospitalized nationally in one month[1]

At one point Bob was in the hospital for a week straight. Shannon and Jeff were exhausted, but one of them was with the baby 24 hours a day. Jeff's employer was very understanding, but there were still times when he needed to go to work. As a result, Shannon often covered the day shift as well as many of the evening and night shifts.

The nurses kept telling her that she didn't have to be there all the time. They encouraged her to go home and rest. She refused, scarcely leaving her baby's side.

She explained, "He was just lying in a crib in a room. They wouldn't necessarily hear him cry. If he needed something, it's not like he could press the call button."

At one point in the grueling ordeal, Shannon looked up to see a nurse enter the room with a syringe full of medicine to inject into Bob's IV. Shannon had noticed that one of his drugs was cloudy and another was clear. One of them filled the syringe completely; the other filled it only a third of the way.

Startled by what she saw in the syringe, she blurted out, "That's three times what he usually gets!"

It was just seconds before the nurse would plunge the needle into the baby's IV. The nurse stopped, looked at her quizzically, and walked out. She returned a moment later, visibly shaken.

Bob was prescribed a large dose of a drug to remove excess fluid from his system and a small dose of a drug to slow his heart rate so that his heart didn't have to work so hard. The nurse had accidentally reversed the doses of the two drugs. She had nearly injected a massive overdose of the heart-slowing drug into his IV. It would have killed him on the spot.

Bob's life was saved only because Shannon wasn't in the bathroom or getting a cup of coffee when the nurse arrived—and because she spoke up.

A week or so later, Shannon took Bob to see a surgeon who was reputed to be the best in the country for pediatric heart problems. He warned her that the posi-

tion of the holes would make it very difficult to operate. But he thought that he might be able to save her son.

Having struggled his entire life—from Easter to the Fourth of July—Bob now lay in one of the best children's hospitals in the country, awaiting open heart surgery. Kept alive only by potent drugs, he was perhaps a week from death. He slept almost all the time now; being awake took too much effort.

Doctor after doctor examined him. Shannon was grateful and encouraged; they were all so attentive to her tiny son. She didn't find out until later that they were doctors in training who were eager to see this critically ill infant because his case was so extreme that it would be a miracle if he survived.

SAD BUT TRUE

1 in 3

Hospital admissions that result in adverse events

Institute for Healthcare Improvement, after studying a sample drawn from records of all adult patients during one month in three hospitals renowned for delivering high-quality care[2]

The day of surgery arrived. The extraordinarily gifted surgeon turned in an astonishing performance, repairing multiple hard-to-reach holes in an organ about the size of a walnut. Bob survived the surgery.

As a result, Jeff and Shannon started to hope that their desperately ill baby might have a shot at a normal life—a chance to see other Easters and other Fourths of July, a chance to see Halloween and Thanksgiving and Christmas.

Bob's experience offers a snapshot of health care in America: catastrophic failures in basic care combined with incredible miracles in high tech, dramatic care. In his case, the miracles won out: today, Bob is an intelligent, active, cheerful child.

Not everyone is so lucky.

Some public figures say that the United States has "the best health care in the world" or even "the best health care system the world has ever known."[3] But this system—despite good intentions—produces a large volume of "adverse events," as mistakes or complications of care are called.

Examples include drug errors, blood clots, infections, severe bedsores, and serious trouble breathing after surgery.[4] Surgeons even "operate on the wrong person or body part as often as 40 times a week."[5]

How To Prevent Hospital Drug Errors

1. **Know what drugs your doctors have ordered**.
   Ask your doctor(s) to tell you the **name**, **strength**, and **timing** for all doses of drugs that you will be given, and write this information down. (*Include IV solutions, injections, pills, liquids, and so forth.*)

2. **Check the drugs brought to you**.
   Each time someone comes into your room to give you a drug, ask its name and the dose, and compare the answers to your list. **If the drug isn't on your list,** or the dosage or timing is different from the doctor's instructions, **decline to take it** until you hear from your doctor(s) that the change is one they authorized.

3. **Track the drugs administered**.
   Write down the name of the drug, the dose given, and the date and time. This step can help you **avoid being double-dosed**. (*For example, sometimes when a shift changes, the new staff don't realize that you were already given your medicine.*)

Excessive bleeding, broken hips from falling when getting out of bed in the hospital, transfusions of the wrong blood type, surgical gear left inside a patient, and dozens of other issues are also seen.[6]

Patients may get the wrong drug, the wrong dose, a drug intended for someone else, a double dose because one care worker doesn't realize that another just gave the patient the prescribed dose, a drug that interacts badly with another, and so forth.

Dr. Jerald Winakur wrote in a prestigious health policy journal:

> **SAD BUT TRUE**
>
> **1**
>
> Number of preventable medication errors that a typical hospital patient is subjected to each day
>
>
>
> Institute of Medicine study, sponsored by the federal Center for Medicare and Medicaid Services[7]

"Three years ago my father, a longtime heart patient, had trouble breathing and complained of chest pain. He was admitted into the hospital with congestive heart failure. This is the hospital in which I have made rounds almost every day for the past three decades. . . . The CEO is my friend and patient. My father's physician is one of my young associates, well-trained and eager. I was confident that my father would receive the best medical care he could get in America today. Yet I would not leave him alone in his hospital room. During the day, if I or my brother or mother could not be there, I had a hired sitter by his bed. . . . It is almost a miracle that any elderly patient gets out of the hospital today relatively unscathed."[8]

Infections

In the mid-1800s, women giving birth died 10-35 percent of the time. In 1847 an Austrian-Hungarian obstetrician, Ignaz Semmelweis, discovered that deaths in hospitals could be cut dramatically if professionals washed their hands and instruments before working on their patients.

Doctors had been coming to attend births straight from performing autopsies, without washing their hands in between, which explained why death rates during childbirth were much higher when doctors attended than when midwives did.

SAD BUT TRUE

3rd

The rank of health care among causes of death in the U.S.

❧

A study in 2000 in *JAMA (Journal of the American Medical Association)* counting only selected problems and thus underestimating deaths due to health care[11]

Doctors took offense at the suggestion that they were responsible. They believed it was simply inevitable that many women would die in childbirth.[9]

Most infections in hospitals today still travel via unwashed hands.[10]

"Christine was a feisty woman!" her husband, Patrick, said fondly. *"She fought for special needs educational plans for families that needed help with their children with the school. She wouldn't be afraid to go in front of a bunch of lawyers and fight it out, or the school principals, or superintendents, or the school board."*

He said, *"I had no chance in an argument with her. We'd argue and she'd be all over me. And finally I would say, 'Whatever you want, honey, it's fine with me. I can't argue with you. You blow me away.' She could argue with the best of them."*

He continued, *"She did a lot of good in her day. She helped a lot of families out that needed it. She would help people get disability payments, people with a lot of medical problems. They would say, 'You're helping my son with the school. Would you help me too?'"*

Patrick talked about their life 20 years earlier, when they were first married. *"She raised horses and was able to walk in the mountains of Colorado, go on hiking trips, and all that."* But Christine had an unusually severe case of scoliosis, and the curve in her back kept getting worse.

"The scoliosis kept slowly crushing her lungs. She lived at home on oxygen, and shortly after that she went into a wheelchair for a couple of years. Eventually she was unable to swallow, and so they had to put a feeding tube in." She also had to have an opening cut in her neck for a tube that allowed air to get into her windpipe (trachea). Christine was 43 years old.

"She fought back. She fought for two years after that. She put up a heck of a fight. She didn't want to die. She was a real fighter. She kept plugging away."

She was in and out of the hospital, and she always had a variety of IV lines—also known as catheters—running into her body. Patrick is philosophical about the infections she got through these IV lines permanently breaching her skin.

"It wasn't so much 'if' they would get infected; it was 'when.' As with any patient in the hospital, they took her temperature a couple of times a day. As soon as she started getting a temperature, that meant that she had an infection. Then they had to pull out the old central line [a type of IV], put in a new one, start an antibiotic, and take care of her that way."

This problem arose so often that Patrick didn't think anything of it when it happened again. But this time the vascular surgeon who had to put in a new IV said that it would have to wait.

"He was very busy and said, 'I can't schedule you for another week or so.' The infection got worse and worse. Eventually, they changed the line, but it was too late. The infection went throughout her body."

> **SAD BUT TRUE**
>
> # 35
>
> Percentage of hospital workers who routinely wash their hands before touching patients
>
>
>
> Dr. Dennis O'Leary, then head of the Joint Commission, which accredits about 19,000 hospitals and other health care organizations in the U.S.[12]

He said somberly, "She was unconscious for a week. She kept dying. Finally, they said to me, 'We worked on her for six hours last night to keep her alive. She's never going to wake up. What do you want to do?' She was going to die anyway. I had to tell them, 'You may as well let her go.'" Christine was 45 years old.

Patrick still feels responsible: "I should have been way more active when I knew she was infected and I knew they were putting it off. I just thought, 'She's made it through so many infections, she'll make it through—it's no big deal.' But she continued to get worse. Then she slipped into a coma. I never should have let that happen. I should have been more proactive. I should have said, 'Get her to another hospital! Do something for her!' I should have been way more assertive than I was, and that's definitely my fault."

Would Christine have died eventually anyway? Yes, as we all will. But she didn't have to die that day.

Researchers have repeatedly found that hospital infections "arise mainly from poor hygiene in hospital procedures, not from how sick patients were when they were admitted."[13]

How To Prevent Hospital Infections

1. **Choose a hospital with lower infection rates.**
   a. Compare infection rates before choosing a hospital, if possible. Search Medicare's **Hospital Compare** site at hospitalcompare.hhs.gov, through this chain of menus:
      >Readmissions, Complications & Deaths
      >Serious Complications and Deaths
      >Serious Complications
      >Get Results for this Hospital
      >Infections from a large venous catheter,
        and bloodstream infection after surgery.
   b. If no information is posted, **ask** the hospital. If you can't get an answer, that's not a good sign.

2. **Ask how the professionals will prevent infections.**
   A good answer about their procedure for inserting major IV lines is, "We use a **checklist.**" A concerning answer is, "We do this all the time; we know what we're doing."

3. **Take steps yourself to prevent infections.**
   a. **Protect the site where any IV line is inserted**—if it gets damp or dirty, ask that the area be cleaned. (*It may be necessary to replace the line with one inserted somewhere else.*)
   b. **Ask everyone** who enters the room—doctors, nurses, aides, clergy, family members, and so forth—**to wash their hands** before approaching the bed.

Research shows that infection rates plummet when a checklist is used to ensure that all the right steps are completed each and every time major IV lines (called "central lines") are inserted.[14]

However, many medical professionals dismiss the idea of using checklists; their stance amounts to, "We do this all the time; we know what we're doing," an approach that results in needless deaths.

Airplane pilots use checklists every single time they prepare to fly, regardless of how experienced they are. The same approach in health care has been shown to save lives.

Dr. Peter Pronovost, a leader in infection control, provides a short checklist for doctors to follow that is proven to prevent such infections:

> **SAD BUT TRUE**
>
> # 75,000
>
> Deaths each year from infections patients get during hospital stays
>
>
>
> The Centers for Disease Control and Prevention, based on a study published in 2014 in the *New England Journal of Medicine* involving 11,282 patients at 182 hospitals[15]

1. Wash your hands.
2. Wear sterile clothing; cover patient with sterile drapes.
3. Avoid putting the catheter [IV line] in the patient's groin, a breeding ground for infection.
4. Clean the patient's skin where the line will go in, using antiseptic.
5. Remove catheters as soon as they are not needed.[16]

Blood Clots

Louise, age 38, had a hysterectomy to eliminate the very heavy bleeding that she had had for years with her menstrual periods. She said, "The attitude from the doctors and nurses was, 'This is routine surgery—a walk in the park.'"

The operation was uneventful, and Louise soon returned home. She does not recall much—if any—discussion about possible complications to watch out for.

Louise said, "One week later, I got up in the morning and had an awful pain in my shoulder when breathing. It was hard to catch my breath. I went back to the surgeon. He said, 'What's wrong with you is a shoulder problem. Go see an orthopedic surgeon.'"

Louise continued, "As the day went on, it got harder and harder to breathe. My friends took me to the hospital. A blood clot had gone through my heart to my lungs."

Louise received emergency treatment and survived. Looking back, she was disturbed that the surgeon immediately assumed that her new problem had nothing to do with the operation he had recently performed.

Many people believe that most blood clots are related to long airplane flights. However, Dr. John A. Heit of the Mayo Clinic noted that more than two-thirds are associated with hospital care.[18] Nearly a third of the people who get blood clots die, typically when a clot breaks off and travels to the lungs, where it interferes with breathing.

Blood clots are more common than heart attacks or strokes and cause more deaths than either of those. Deaths from blood clots are expected to increase: older people are at greater risk, and the population is aging.[19]

Medicare, the federal health insurance program for the elderly and disabled, often won't pay hospitals for treating blood clots related to inpatient care, because they are considered completely preventable.[20]

Despite these facts, most people have no idea that they are at risk, and they often aren't screened or treated to prevent clots in the hospital.

As was true in Louise's case, blood clots may not become evident until the patient is home. At that point, people may let down their guard, assuming that any risks from hospital care ended when they drove out of the hospital parking lot.

Dr. Joseph A. Caprini at Northwestern University has developed a model to assess a patient's risk of developing a blood clot. It assigns points to each of about two dozen risk factors, such as age, surgery that lasts 45 minutes or more, obesity, smoking, and recent bone fractures.[21]

How To Prevent Hospital Blood Clots

1. **Find out your risk.**
    Before a hospital stay, use the **Risk Assessment Tool** found at http://www.clotcare.com/dvtriskassessmenttool. pdf to get a rough idea of your risk level for blood clots.

2. **Get a prevention plan.**
    a. **Review the results** of your risk assessment with your doctor, and ask what steps will be taken so that you don't get blood clots.
    b. Ensure that the plan is put into **action.**

3. **Watch for symptoms.**
    Both in the hospital and after you leave, **get immediate attention** if you have any of the following **unexplained symptoms**, or others as advised by your doctor:
    a. Sudden onset of **shortness of breath.**
    b. **Chest pain** or discomfort that worsens when you take a deep breath or cough.
    c. **Lightheadedness**, dizziness, or fainting.
    d. **Rapid pulse.**
    e. **Sweating.**
    f. **Coughing up blood.**
    g. **Anxiety** or nervousness.
    h. **Swelling or pain** in a leg, ankle, or foot (*may start in the calf; may feel like cramping or a charley horse*).
    i. **Warmth** in area of swelling or pain.
    j. **Changes in skin color** (*turning pale, red, or blue*).[22]

Consider a 55-year-old woman who has just had surgery lasting an hour to treat a broken hip. She scores one point for her age, five points for her broken hip, and two points for the 60-minute surgery, for a total of eight points. Of the people who score five or more points, 40-80 percent develop blood clots.[23]

Several approaches to prevention are common. Drugs that thin the blood can help prevent clots from forming. A compression device can repeatedly squeeze patients' lower legs while they are confined to bed. People can be helped out of bed to move around as soon as possible after surgery.[25]

Expected Harm

Doctors sometimes act as if side effects and complications appear out of nowhere: unfortunate, unpredictable, and unavoidable accidents, unrelated to the care they provide. They may simply shrug in the face of overwhelming evidence that the care they give may kill or injure many people each year—even though many of the problems could easily be prevented.

One doctor said, "As long as it doesn't go beyond the [national average] published error rate, I'm fine." Another said, "We're like lawyers. We just provide services by the hour and sometimes it works and sometimes it doesn't." Doctors too frequently view preventable problems as inevitable, a stance that ethics experts call "moral disengagement."[26]

Daniel Levinson, the inspector general of the United States Department of Health & Human Services, noted that hospitals are required by the federal government to track, analyze, and report mistakes and other adverse events that hurt patients.

However, hospital workers report only about one mistake out of every seven. When asked why they didn't report problems, they offered inspectors the following explanations:

- They didn't realize that people had been hurt.
- They thought the harm was normal for hospital patients.
- They thought it was someone else's job to report mistakes.
- They thought the problem was so common that it didn't need to be reported.
- They thought the problem was so rare that it didn't need to be reported.[27]

SAD BUT TRUE

42nd

Rank order of life expectancy in the United States compared to 222 other countries

The United States Central Intelligence Agency World Factbook in 2014[28]

Why is there so little focus on this issue? Leadership is responsible. Hospital boards set the priorities for the hospital. They tell the CEO what he has to do well for them to be happy with his work; they decide if he may keep his job and how big a raise he gets. Only half the leaders of hospital boards said that quality of care was one of their top two priorities.[29]

The federal government is working on a system to allow patients themselves to report medical errors and unsafe practices.[30]

While there are pockets of improvement and some truly inspired initiatives,[31] results overall are weak. One article written in 2005, reporting little or no improvement from five years earlier, was titled, "To Err Is Human; To Fail to Improve Is Unconscionable."[32]

Four years after that, in 2009, the government concluded that the situation was actually getting worse.[33] In 2011, a cover story in a major health journal reported that problems in hospitals "may be ten times greater than previously measured."[34]

What's the best way to protect yourself if you must go to the hospital? One step is have a friend, family member, or other trusted individual with you at all times to act as your advocate, taking notes and asking questions. To cover all the hours in a day, you may need several people to help.

The next three pages offer steps to take to gain access for your advocate, be an effective advocate, and get urgently needed help in the hospital.

How To Get Access for Your Advocate

1. **Learn your rights.**
   See **A Patient's Guide to the HIPAA Privacy Rule**: When Health Care Providers May Communicate about You with Your Family, Friends, or Others Involved In Your Care, which can be found at: http://www.hhs.gov/ocr/privacy/hipaa/understanding/consumers/consumer_ffg.pdf. *(Sometimes, doctors and nurses say that HIPAA prevents them from talking with your family or friends. That statement usually is not accurate. The information in this brochure can help you counter that claim.)*

2. **Explain your intentions ahead of time, if possible.**
   Explain to your doctor and the hospital before you are admitted that you would like **specific people you identify** to be able to see your chart, ask questions, and get information from the doctors and nurses taking care of you.

3. **Get the paperwork done.**
   Ask if you need to **sign a HIPAA release** or waiver. HIPAA *(Health Insurance Portability and Accountability Act of 1996)* protects the privacy of your medical information.

How To Be an Effective Advocate

1. **Track important information in a notebook.**
   a. **Doctors**: contact information for the patient's primary care doctor, for all the doctors involved in this hospital visit, and for the "attending physician," who is in charge of the patient's overall care in the hospital.
   b. **Other sources of help**: contact information for the hospital's Patient Relations department, Patient Ombudsman, and/or Rapid Response Team.
   c. **Tests and treatments ordered**: for drugs, note the name of the drug, the dosage, and how often the patient is expected to get it.
   d. **Tests and treatments the patient actually gets**.
   e. **Questions, concerns, or observations**.
   f. **Conversations** with key medical personnel (*e.g., topics discussed, next steps*).

2. **Act for the patient with medical personnel.**
   a. Share important observations and **ask questions** (*prompted by notes in the notebook*). Be polite but assertive. Write down answers or responses.
   b. **Verify** that **tests and treatments** about to be delivered are ones ordered.
   c. **Ask for a nutritionist's evaluation** if the patient eats or drinks little.
   d. **Use "How To" guides** in this book to help prevent **infections** (*p. 8*), **blood clots** (*p. 11*), **delirium** (*p. 26*), and **bedsores** (*p. 68*).

3. **Help the patient cope with being in the hospital.**
   a. Make sure the **call button** is in reach.
   b. Help with **eyeglasses** and/or **hearing aids**.
   c. Provide **companionship** (*even if simply a silent, comforting presence*).

4. **Get help if the patient suddenly seems worse.**

How To Get Urgently Needed Help

1. **Talk to the right caregivers: doctors and nurses.**
   a. It will not help if you talk only to someone who picks up menus or takes people for tests.
   b. **Remain calm** and non-threatening.
   c. Explain that you urgently need to speak with whoever is **in charge of this patient** at this moment.

2. **Explain clearly and concisely what is wrong.**
   a. Be as **specific** as possible.
   b. Explain why you are **concerned**.

3. **Escalate, if urgent problems aren't addressed.**
   a. Go up the **chain of command**. Ask to speak to the "**nurse supervisor**" or the "**attending physician**."
   b. Contact the **Rapid Response Team** or **Patient Ombudsman**, if the hospital has such a function.

4. **Try other routes, if none of the above works.**
   a. Ask to speak to the **most senior member of the hospital staff available**. (*This will be an executive who may or may not be a doctor, but who knows exactly how the hospital works.*)
   b. Try calling the patient's **primary care doctor**, who may be able to elicit action from other health care professionals when you can't.
   c. Try speaking to a manager in the hospital's **Risk Management department**, which wants to ensure good patient care to reduce the risk of lawsuits. You might also try the **Quality Control** or **Quality improvement** department.

Health care also harms people outside of hospitals, according to a study in *JAMA*, the *Journal of the American Medical Association*. This harm is more likely to result from misdiagnosis than from surgical mishaps, but damage may be as common and as serious.[35]

Despite all the evidence, doctors, nurses, and other health care professionals sometimes do not see problems because they are not looking for them, misled by the dangerous assumption that we have the best health care in the world.

In Hans Christian Andersen's fairy tale *The Emperor's New Clothes*, the townspeople didn't believe what they themselves saw. They were told that only very smart people could see the emperor's fine new clothes as he paraded down the street.

When they looked at the naked emperor, they were embarrassed. They assumed that everyone else could see the suit. Since they didn't want to appear stupid, they just agreed that the suit was very fine. It took a child who relied on his own senses instead of succumbing to social pressure to break the spell.

Health care in America has something in common with *The Emperor's New Clothes*. The health care system is not what you've been led to believe it is. You can break the spell. You can discover how to overcome dangerous assumptions that may threaten the health—and even the lives—of you, your family, and your friends.

SAD BUT TRUE

98

Percentage of the time that hospitals, having identified a problem that hurt a patient, failed to make changes to avoid similar harm in the future

※

Inspector General of the U.S. Department of Health & Human Services in 2012, in a study of 293 incidents of patient harm across 189 hospitals; in 288 cases, no changes were made[36]

2

"You'll be fine once the doctor patches you up"

Doctors focus on handling the immediate crisis, rather than on what will happen once the patient goes home. As a result, some side effects and complications fly under the radar screen. Tragically, however, lives are needlessly ruined when easily preventable complications are allowed to take root.

Short hospital stay, permanent harm

Mildred and George, both in their 80's, lived in their own apartment in a retirement community that I'll call Pine Lakes. Mildred had been a professor of art history at a state university, and George had been an executive with an import/export company. They had enjoyed traveling all over the world.

Now, Mildred and George were having trouble managing their finances and preparing their meals, but they treasured their independence. Mildred loved their home, particularly the sun porch opening onto a greenbelt. She spent hours there, enjoying the bright colors and appealing scents of the flowers, the songs of the birds, the green leaves rustling in the breeze, and the fluffy white clouds against the blue sky.

One night, their daughter Carol's phone rang around 9:30 p.m. Caller ID showed that the call came from Pine Lakes, but not from her parents' apartment. Before she even picked up the phone, Carol felt a sense of dread. The caller was a nurse in the health center.

SAD BUT TRUE

60

Percentage of patients ages 40-60 who become delirious in the hospital

Dr. Wes Ely, founder of the Vanderbilt ICU Delirium and Cognitive Impairment Study Group located at Vanderbilt University[37]

"Your mother fell in her living room. She is in an ambulance on her way to the hospital to be evaluated for a possible broken hip."

"Oh, no!" Carol said. This, she thought, is the beginning of the end.

She threw a couple changes of clothes into a bag and arrived at the sprawling hospital two hours later. By 1:00 a.m., doctors confirmed that Mildred had shattered her hip.

Two days later, Mildred said fretfully, "I don't see why I can't join the family out on the patio. Everybody is out there. I can hear them. Why do I have to stay inside?"

"Mom," Carol said carefully, "You are in the hospital. You broke your hip. You had surgery yesterday to replace your hip joint. The people you hear outside the door are hospital employees. This isn't the family reunion at my house. That was two months ago."

"But I just want to be with the family. I don't see what harm it will cause if I go outside to be with the family for just a little while."

Carol distracted her mother by talking about her children.

Then Mildred asked, "Why am I in a hallway? Why am I lying in a hallway?"

"You're not in a hallway, Mom. You're in a hospital room."

"No, I'm not. See all the people walking by?"

Carol kept trying, saying, "Mom, those are people coming to visit the woman in the bed by the window. You're not in a hallway."

"I don't want to be lying in a hallway."

The next time she saw Mildred's doctor, Carol said, "She's irrational. She keeps trying to fold the sheet she's lying under so she can put it away 'upstairs in the linen closet.' She hasn't lived any place with an upstairs for seven years. She thinks the television set is a window. She thinks it's night all the time because the TV screen is dark, since the TV is turned off. What's happening?"

"Oh, don't worry," the doctor assured her. "That's completely normal. It happens to everybody. It's disorienting to be in the hospital. As soon as we can get her back to Pine Lakes, she'll be fine."[38]

Three days after surgery, an ambulance took Mildred back to Pine Lakes, where she was settled into a bed in the skilled nursing unit.

Two months after the operation, Carol took her mother to see the surgeon. Mildred had healed well and did not limp or have any pain. The surgeon examined Mildred and watched her walk.

"This is astonishing!" the surgeon said. "She's doing as well after eight weeks as I had hoped she might be doing after twelve weeks!"

Relieved by the surgeon's good report, Carol arranged to meet with the nurse in charge of Mildred's care.

She asked, "How soon can my mother return to her apartment?"

The nurse said, "She's never going back."

"What? What do you mean?"

"As far as her hip goes, she could go back now," the nurse said. "She could have gone back weeks ago. But cognitively, she's got some big problems. She needs constant help remembering how to do everything—get dressed, find the dining area, everything. She's never going to leave skilled nursing."

"But she was living in her own apartment! Maybe she needs to be in assisted living, but not skilled nursing!"

The nurse was unmoved. "I didn't know her before she came here. I'm basing my conclusions on what I see of her here. And she isn't going anywhere."

Mildred was inconsolable when she understood that her apartment was lost to her forever. The staff said that she would adjust in a few weeks, but she didn't. She asked about the apartment every day for months and tried to figure out how to find her way back to it whenever she was outside.

She often sat silently in the dark for hours, lights off and shades drawn. Eventually, the staff realized the depth of her despair and treated her for depression. With time, Mildred recovered her good spirits--but not her mental faculties.

Carol told her family, "I think Mom lost about half her mental capacity when she was in the hospital. At first, they told me that it was the result of the anesthesia and the painkillers, and that it would take quite a while for those to clear out of her system. But it's been months."

SAD BUT TRUE

66-84

Percentage of hospital patients whose delirium is not diagnosed and therefore not treated

Dr. Wes Ely, Vanderbilt University, based on a number of research studies[39]

SAD BUT TRUE

30

Seconds it typically takes to diagnose delirium, using a simple checklist; sadly, although it is easy to do, it is usually not done

Dr. Wes Ely, expert in delirium, Vanderbilt University[40]

Mildred is still living in skilled nursing, seven years after breaking her hip. The few days of delirium she experienced in the hospital led directly to long-term cognitive impairment. If she hadn't had delirium, she would have ended up in assisted living.

In her retirement community, assisted living apartments each have a balcony or patio looking out onto the greenbelt, allowing residents to sit and enjoy the sights, sounds, and scents of nature. The apartments also offer four times as much space as skilled nursing.

In assisted living, residents have more privacy, the option to keep more of their furniture and belongings, more engaging company, more interesting activities, and more freedom.

But Mildred didn't get a chance to lead that richer life. Instead, she is spending her final years in a small room in an institution where alarms clamor every few minutes. She doesn't have a porch, patio, or balcony where she can sit and commune with nature. She has one window. It overlooks the parking lot.

Delirium

Where would you find an environment with the following characteristics?

- Individuals' clothing and other personal belongings are removed.
- They have little information about, or control over, what is happening to them or around them.
- They are in pain and are physically restrained.
- They are subjected to bright lights shining on them 24/7.
- They can't get away from frequent, loud, jarring noises that sound at unpredictable intervals around the clock.
- They rapidly become so sleep deprived and disoriented that they can't tell if it is day or night.

Every audience asked to name a site with these characteristics has given the same two correct answers: a prison camp for terrorist suspects—and a hospital ICU (Intensive Care Unit).[41]

People in an ICU also have two big handicaps that prisoners usually do not. First, they are very sick. Second, they are typically drugged.[42] About two-thirds of them develop delirium.[43]

Delirium can develop in a few hours. People who are delirious "cannot think clearly, have trouble paying attention, have a hard time understanding what is going on around them, [and] may see or hear things that are not there."[45] The hallucinations are very convincing to the patients.

People who are older, sicker, and/

SAD BUT TRUE

10

Years of immediate and permanent mental decline that older people may experience due to a few days of untreated hospital-induced delirium

❧

Research involving 1,335 patients followed for up to 13 years, published in the medical journal *Neurology* in 2012 and described in the *New York Times*[44]

or more heavily medicated are more likely to develop delirium. Commonly prescribed drugs called benzodiazepines increase the risk. A subset including Versed triples the risk of delirium, and some doses of some drugs, including Ativan, almost guarantee it.[46]

Doctors and nurses often keep patients heavily sedated to minimize pain. But many such patients experience horrific nightmares and hallucinations that may feature gory images and the belief that they are prisoners. It's an understandable mistake for very stressed minds to make: patients are usually tethered to machines and may be immobilized by sedatives. Their minds try to make sense of their inability to move.[47]

Many hospital patients develop delirium even if, like Mildred, they aren't in the ICU. The most troublesome problems with delirium may surface after a hospital stay. Survivors of even a few days of delirium often experience serious long-term problems such as post-traumatic stress disorder and/or permanent cognitive decline.[48] Like Mildred, they may never go home again.[49]

SAD BUT TRUE

50

Percentage reduction in delirium among ICU patients given earplugs so they could sleep, compared to other similar ICU patients not given earplugs; sadly, very few patients are ever given earplugs

❀

Study of 136 patients reported in the medical journal *Critical Care* in 2012[51]

Delirium is considered easy to prevent,[50] and actions required to do so do not interfere with medical treatment. One simple example is that dimming the lights at night goes a long way toward keeping people oriented.

Some hospitals have made changes to reduce delirium. However, according to Dr. Wes Ely, founder of Vanderbilt University's ICU Delirium and Cognitive Impairment Study Group, simple action steps needed are typically not taken.

The health care system assumes that recovery is all but assured when doctors put down their scalpels or prescription pads. As a result, signs heralding long-term harm can be easy to see and still not register with doctors and nurses. That seems to be one reason that delirium isn't noticed or addressed in most hospital patients who experience it.

A questionnaire can be used to diagnose delirium very quickly. Found at http://www.icudelirium.org/docs/CAM_ICU_worksheet.pdf, the form includes simple questions that doctors and nurses ask the patient. Examples are, "Will a stone float on water?" and "Does one pound weigh more than two pounds?" The patient is also asked to follow simple instructions such as, "Hold up this many fingers," while the tester holds up two fingers.

Even if the patient appears unresponsive, taking steps to prevent (and even to treat) delirium can help avoid the tragic loss of independence that too often results from this complication of hospital care.

The boxes on the next two pages offer action steps doctors and nurses (health care professionals) and family and friends (advocates) can take to prevent and address delirium.

How Professionals Can Address Delirium

1. **Repeatedly check the patient's mental status.**
   a. Assess and document the patient's mental status **every 4-6 hours**.
   b. Bring patients on ventilators **out of the sedation fog** at frequent intervals, to check their mental status and ability to breathe on their own.

2. **Reduce or eliminate causes of delirium related to treatment and to the hospital environment.**
   a. **Sedation**: reduce it to a minimum.
   b. **Immobility**: as soon as possible, remove physical restraints and medical equipment that restricts motion, provide range of motion exercises, and get patients up and moving.
   c. **Sleep deprivation**: provide earplugs and eye masks, dim the lights at night, and reduce or eliminate loud noises, alarms, and other disruptions.
   d. **Disorientation**: repeatedly remind patients where they are, and explain clearly what is happening to them.
   e. **Dehydration** and **malnutrition**: ensure that patients get enough fluids and nourishment.

3. **Address promptly any medical causes of delirium.**
   a. Control **blood sugar**.
   b. Address **electrolyte imbalances**.
   c. Treat **infections**.

4. **Encourage patients to engage.**
   a. Make available their **eyeglasses/hearing aids/other devices**.
   b. Provide **mentally stimulating activities** several times a day.

How You Can Address Delirium

1. **Learn more about delirium.**
   This background will enable you to have useful conversations with the patient's doctor. See http://www.icudeliri-
   um.org/docs/delirium_education_brochure.pdf.

2. **Work with the professionals.**
   a. Watch for behavior or thinking that is not normal for
      the patient, and ask to have such **incidents noted in
      the patient's chart**.
   b. **Ask how the cause** of the patient's altered mental
      state **will be identified and addressed**.
   c. **Follow up** to ensure that needed steps are taken,
      including the simplest ones of dimming the lights and
      providing earplugs at night.

3. **Help patients engage.**
   a. Make sure that patients have their **eyeglasses** or
      hearing aids. Bring cases for these, labeled with the
      patient's name and the intended contents, so that the
      devices can be properly stored when the patient isn't
      wearing them. (*Otherwise, it is easy for them to get lost.*)
   b. Share favorite **photographs**, **music**, and **TV or radio
      programs**, as circumstances permit.
   c. **Talk** about familiar people and activities.
   d. **Explain what is happening** to them.

Continuing treatment long after a hospital stay

Robert was smart, friendly, and a joy to be around. The former owner of a small family business, he spent hours every day reading. His mind was razor-sharp. When he was 85, he was admitted to the hospital as a result of a mini-stroke, and he was prescribed a blood thinner.

His hospital stay was uneventful and he was soon home, taking the blood thinner as directed. Life went on much as it had before.

One day two or three months later, his wife Joan was driving them home from her 50th college reunion. She was startled when all of a sudden Robert cried out, "My eyes! My eyes! Something terrible is happening!"

Within minutes, he was blind—totally and permanently blind.

Joan explained, "His retinas exploded with massive bleeding. Within the next five hours, his three doctors—his eye doctor, his general practitioner, and his heart doctor—all said, 'Take him off the blood thinner!'" Robert's several medical problems, including a chronic eye disease and diabetes, had increased his risk of bleeding and blindness as a result of taking the drug.

Joan said, "When I asked the eye doctor why no one told us about these risks, he said, 'Well, most people would rather be alive and blind than dead.'"

Joan was appalled and furious: "When the patient is 85, don't you think you should give him that choice?"

She recalled, "I was shocked when I found out two facts. First, his three doctors had never talked to each other. Second, the general practitioner and the eye doctor both knew that the cardiologist had prescribed the blood thinner, but they didn't say anything. I often wonder how different our outcome would have been if Robert's eye doctor had spoken up. What if the eye doctor had said to the cardiologist, 'Take Robert off the blood thinner as soon as the crisis has passed'? Would the last six years of his life have been different? Given an option, Robert would have chosen to die at 85 rather than live to 91 totally blind—reading was his life."

It is worth noting that Robert had been almost completely deaf for many years before his mini-stroke. Hearing aids did not help.

Joan said, "When he went blind, he was almost entirely cut off from the world. In minutes, he lost the ability to interact with the world of ideas. And that's how he spent the last six years of his life."

How To Improve Care Coordination

1. **Get information.**
    a. Read **Hospital Discharge Planning**: A Guide for Families and Caregivers, at http://caregiver.org/hospital-discharge-planning-guide-families-and-caregivers.
    b. Get more suggestions and **checklists** at http://www.caretransitions.org, the website of the Care Transitions Program.

2. **Get personalized help.**
    a. Take advantage of guidance offered by **transitions coaches**, transitional care nurses, or other experts in care transitions provided by your hospital or insurance plan.
    b. Pay attention to **advice they offer** about how to manage your medicines and follow-up care, know if a serious problem is developing, and capture basic information about your health conditions and treatment plans.
    c. Find out if your insurance will provide **visiting nurses or occupational therapists** for a few visits to help you in your home.

3. **Help doctors focus.**
    a. Tell every doctor at every visit **all major medical conditions you have**, and ask specifically how any new treatment proposed might worsen your health given those other conditions.
    b. Remind your doctor **what you most care about being able to do**, and ask if the new treatment is likely to make those activities easier or harder.

Lack of a stable state

How you fare after you are discharged may depend as much on what happens at home as it does on what happened in the hospital. Yet at home you may be on your own, without professionals to help you or provide detailed guidance. Maybe treatments started in the hospital should be continued at home. Maybe not. Who has enough information to decide?

Typically, primary care doctors don't even get reports about their patients' hospital stays before they see them the first time after they are discharged—and when they do, the reports often leave out critical information, such as test results, medicines prescribed, and plans for follow-up.[52]

In Robert's case, all the doctors had all the relevant information, but they failed to reevaluate him. Continuing with the treatment months later put him in a dangerous and unstable condition. But he didn't know that.

See the previous page for steps to take to improve care coordination.

One box unchecked

Linda[53] and Greg are both intelligent, articulate, and retired. They have a lovely home in a pleasant neighborhood where they had always enjoyed taking long walks. But then Linda developed an unexplained infection in her knee that required emergency surgery to treat. She then developed sepsis, a life-threatening complication. Her care was further complicated because she had diabetes and a chronic heart condition.

She spent time in the ICU (Intensive Care Unit), and it was cause for celebration when she was deemed to be well enough to be transferred to a regular hospital room. Then she was sent to a skilled nursing facility to recuperate further.

The care there did not meet her needs, and when her husband Greg was sitting with her one day, she turned to him in desperation and said, "Help me. I just can't breathe. I really can't breathe." Greg leapt up and went running down the hall to get help. Twenty minutes later, an ambulance arrived. Linda was admitted to the hospital after frenzied treatment in the emergency room to save her life.

After that stay, she spent about three weeks in a specialized rehabilitation hospital, where she made a slow but steady recovery. Finally, she was considered well enough to go home. Grateful that she had survived, Greg was very thoughtful and thorough in making arrangements for her care at home.

Linda needed help with both medical issues and personal care, and the agency they contacted sent a nurse to evaluate her needs. Then the nurse came for an hour or two a few times a week, and oversaw an aide who helped Linda with tasks that can be hard to manage when you've been very sick, such as taking a shower. Care got off to a promising start. Then disaster struck.

Linda reported, "Two weeks later, an aide came in to help me take a shower. I was really unsteady on my feet, and she had to be with me the whole time. It was the first time she'd come to do that. I went to get into the shower."

Greg had carefully installed a bench and grab bars in the shower before Linda had come home. But because of the layout of the shower, the grab bars had to be at the back, out of her reach as she entered. The aide had not brought any equipment to use to help ensure that Linda did not fall.

Linda said, "I stepped into the shower, and my foot went out on me. I fell and went into the corner of the shower. There was no room for the other leg, and it snapped. I was lying there and the aide called 911. The next thing I know, there are six EMTs standing over me, discussing how they are going to get me up."

How could care go so wrong?

Linda's husband Greg offered one answer: "I requested all of her records from the home health agency. One thing I noticed in there was that one of the questions they ask [on the evaluation form used by the nurse who assessed Linda before the agency started providing services] is whether this patient is at risk of falling. They did not have that checked off, so from the nurse's perspective, she was not at risk of falling. I think that was an error. She'd just had knee surgery."

Linda had also just been in the hospital and other advanced care settings for roughly six weeks, suggesting that she was likely to be weaker than normal.

She added, "Also, I had been diagnosed with congestive heart failure," some symptoms of which are dizziness, fatigue, and weakness. Further, she was 68 years old, meaning that she had a higher risk of falling than would a similar individual a decade or two younger.

Because the agency had not recorded that Linda was at risk of falling, they would not have instructed the aide to take special precautions in helping Linda with her shower. This one tiny error caused devastating and permanent harm.

Linda developed another massive infection in the leg that broke. Extensive surgery was required to remove infected tissue. She didn't respond well to the antibiotics, and it seemed as if the large surgical wound would never heal.

About 2-1/2 years after her saga started, Linda said, "I am still in a wheelchair."

If you evaluate each medical incident individually, in all but a few cases, Linda received outstanding care. She was treated at a regular hospital in five emergency room visits and four hospital stays, at a rehabilitation hospital two different times, in two different skilled nursing facilities, in an outpatient physical therapy clinic, and at a specialized wound care clinic. She received care at home from two different home health agencies, one of them for two different periods.

The causes of her infections are unknown, so one cannot say if they resulted from substandard care. Based on the available information about everything else that happened, the quality of care Linda got appears to be well above average, with the exception of one stay in a skilled nursing facility and one assisted shower at home.

And yet, she is still in a wheelchair.

Most of Linda's problems would have been avoided if the nurse had checked the box identifying Linda as at risk for falls. Doing so would have triggered precautions that would almost certainly have prevented her fall in the shower.

That simple change would have saved hundreds of thousands of dollars, avoided about ten months of extensive medical care, and almost certainly left Linda with no need for a wheelchair.

SAD BUT TRUE

34

Percentage of Medicare patients who are readmitted to the hospital within 90 days, often because of gaps in the transition between the hospital and home

Study in the *New England Journal of Medicine* of nearly 12 million hospitalizations among Medicare patients over two years[54]

Linda's experience provides some insight into a puzzling paradox. We have the best medical technology in the world and a highly competent, well trained work force. We spend more money per person on health care than any other country does, by a wide margin. Yet highly respected research reveals that health care in America unintentionally kills hundreds of thousands of people a year and injures millions more—leaving many of them, like Linda, permanently disabled. How can both sets of facts be true?

One reason they are both true is that care is typically not coordinated well between sites. Details are often lost in translation during "care transitions," which are moves from one site to another, such as hospital to rehabilitation facility, or hospital to home. Inadequate thought may go into planning such transfers. Many people end up back in the hospital in short order, and most of these readmissions appear to be preventable.[55]

On the next two pages, see questions to ask before leaving the hospital.

What To Ask Before Leaving the Hospital

1. **Basics**
    a. **When am I leaving** the hospital?
    b. **Where am I going** (*home, rehab center*)?
    c. **Who is taking me** there?
    d. **What are all my diagnoses** (*the medical problems that put or kept me in the hospital*)?

2. **Emergencies**
    a. What **symptoms** would suggest a serious problem?
    b. **Who/what number would I call?** Is it different at night or on weekends?

3. **Medicines**
    a. What is the **name and purpose** of each drug prescribed as I leave the hospital?
    b. How will the prescriptions get **filled**?
    c. Am I to keep taking the **drugs I was taking before** I came to the hospital?
    d. What is my **daily medication schedule**—which drugs/how much/when?
    e. Should I **renew the hospital prescriptions** when they run out? Restart medicines I had been taking before? Neither?

4. **In-home help**
    a. Have **arrangements** been made for people to come to the house to help me?
    b. **Who** is coming (*or name of agency*)?
    c. **When** will they come?
    d. **What** will they do for me?
    e. How do I **get in touch** with them?
    f. How will they **get all the information** about me and my hospital stay that they need to safely care for me?
    g. What **backup plans** are in place in case helpers don't show up?

What To Ask Before Leaving the Hospital, cont.

5. **Daily activities**
    a. What **special arrangements** do I need (*such as a raised toilet seat after hip replacement*)? Who has **taken care of** them?
    b. Am I at **risk for falls**? What **precautions** are needed when I stand, walk, use the toilet/shower/bath, dress/undress, and go up/down stairs?
    c. **How much fluid** do I need to drink? (*Dehydration can lead to serious complications.*)
    d. **How will I get meals** if I am too weak to open food containers or run a microwave?
    e. When can I resume **normal activities**? (*When is it safe to climb the stairs, drive, and so forth?*)

6. **Supplies and equipment**
    a. **What supplies do I need**, such as oxygen, a hospital bed, a bedside commode, specific bandages, or assistive devices such as a walker?
    b. **How will I get them**, particularly if I am discharged on Friday or over the weekend?
    c. Who will **receive** them, **set them up**, and **teach me** how to use them?

7. **Follow-ups**
    a. What **doctor** is in charge of my care once I leave the hospital?
    b. What **test results** are still expected? How, when, and from whom will I get them?
    c. Which doctors do I need to see after I leave? How soon? Are **appointments** scheduled?
    d. How/when will those doctors **get all the information** about my hospital stay that they need to oversee my care?

The hospital will not be able to answer all the questions on the preceding two pages. Family members, friends, and/or paid caregivers may need to be involved.

Efforts are underway to help people close some of these gaps when they leave the hospital. The Care Transitions program developed by Dr. Eric Coleman, who heads the Division of Health Care Policy and Research at the University of Colorado's medical school, trains transitions coaches who help patients understand their conditions, their medicines, actions they need to take, and so forth.

The program has been implemented in many places across the country, but there are still thousands of hospitals and insurers that do not participate. See caretransitions.org, which offers resources for patients and their family members as well as for professionals.

A similar program, called the Transitional Care Model at www.transitionalcare.info, was designed by Mary Naylor, a professor at the University of Pennsylvania School of Nursing and the director of New Courtland Center for Transitions and Health.

Don't hesitate to accept any such services offered by your hospital or insurer; the help you receive can make a big difference in your recovery.

3

"Side effects are no big deal"

Drugs, surgery, and other treatments are powerful tools that can and do save lives every day. But they also harbor hidden dangers. If you run across someone brandishing a gun in a dark alley at midnight, you know that you're in trouble. If you see ads full of smiling people whose lives reportedly have improved because of a medical treatment, you might not realize that such treatments can also cause serious harm.

Too many drugs

When Alesandra's doctor tore a sheet off the prescription pad and handed it to her at the end of her annual check-up, Alesandra never imagined that it would launch a 10-year nightmare—one that she would be lucky to survive.

Alesandra, age 35, was quite healthy before that doctor's visit. She didn't take any medicine, and she didn't smoke or drink. She ran the western divisions for an engineering firm. Based in San Diego, she traveled worldwide, handling clients all over the globe.

"I was successful. I was doing quite well," Alesandra reported.

That life ended with her annual check-up. When her doctor asked if she had any complaints, Alesandra mentioned as an afterthought that she was having trouble sleeping, almost certainly due to a family problem that would be resolved shortly.

SAD BUT TRUE

89

Percentage of patients who were not alerted to possible side effects by their doctors

❀

Mayo Clinic study of 172 patients given new prescriptions when they left the hospital[56]

Her doctor didn't even ask if Alesandra wanted a drug to help her sleep; she just gave her a prescription. Always one to follow the rules, Alesandra obediently stood in line at the pharmacy to get the bottle of pills and started taking them as prescribed.

Soon, Alesandra recalled, "Everything began to come apart."

She thought it strange when she developed bronchitis a few weeks after her check-up, because she never got sick. She didn't learn until years later that lung problems are a known side effect of the sleeping pills.

After taking a potent antibiotic to treat the bronchitis, she developed bizarre heart arrhythmias, a condition that was treated with more drugs.

And so it went, for ten years.

Because she typically didn't develop new symptoms until a few weeks after she started taking a new medicine, Alesandra didn't realize that the drugs were causing the problems. She was sent to one specialist after another. A model patient, she told every doctor about all the other doctors she was seeing and about all the drugs she was taking.

None of her doctors commented on the lengthy and always growing list of medicines. None of them mentioned that the many drugs might be hurting her more than helping her. Each treated the latest problem as if it were the only medical issue she had. And they simply wrote more prescriptions for more drugs.

Eventually, Alesandra was taking more than 30 pills a day—nearly 12,000 pills a year. She suffered from seizures, lung infections, breathing problems that landed her in the emergency room, repeated urinary tract infections, weakness in her legs, an uneven gait, severe ankle sprains, and intense back pain. Ironically, her insomnia—the problem for which the first drug was prescribed—worsened.

No longer able to work, Alesandra lived on disability checks. She suffered from depression as her world shrank until it was filled only with medical problems, doctors' appointments, and drugs.

She commented, "There was never any discussion about getting off the drugs. There was no exit strategy."

Once, the psychiatrist treating her depression mentioned that a drug company was paying for his family's vacation to Germany. Alesandra reported ruefully that she didn't think anything about it at the time—even as he handed her a new prescription for one of that company's drugs.

One day, she rebelled. Through an excruciating process that she wouldn't recommend to anyone, she stopped taking all the drugs in very short order.

She said, "I am nearly 54. I am perfectly healthy. I can walk fine. I have no pain. Today I am not on any medicines, just nutrients and good food and exercise." She co-founded Point of Return (pointofreturn.com) to help others prescribed a high volume of drugs.

SAD BUT TRUE

1 in 4

Patients who experienced side effects within 3 months of starting a new medicine

Study of 1,202 patients in 4 medical practices, reported in the *New England Journal of Medicine*[57]

Although Alesandra survived, she lost ten years of her life to polypharmacy, the prescribing of (too) many drugs for one person.

Lawrence, age 67, had a different experience: even one drug was too many.

Lawrence was newly retired from his job as a high school principal in New Mexico when he landed in the hospital with a heart attack. His doctors put him on a drug to control cholesterol. He continued taking the medicine after he got out of the hospital, and he felt lucky to be alive.

Four years later, his health took a turn for the worse. He developed a rash all over his body. He saw doctor after doctor, all of whom found his symptoms quite puzzling. Eventually, his dermatologist referred him to a nationally renowned clinic where he underwent days of testing. They ruled out skin cancer, lupus, Lyme disease, and every other serious condition they could think of.

Three years after that, Lawrence became very ill.

He noted, "I began to feel body aches and a sick feeling in my digestive system." Very soon, "the onset of pain and weakness caused me to seek out a new family doctor. When he saw my blood tests he immediately discovered my liver was almost destroyed and muscle structure profoundly impaired."

Fortunately for Lawrence, the doctor quickly ordered him to stop taking the

cholesterol medicine that he had been on for seven years. He also prescribed a fat-free diet and almost complete rest.

Lawrence said somberly, "I realize he saved my life. We have since heard of others who did not recover, but died by letting this go on too long."

The next three months, Lawrence reports, "were utter agony." He was unable to bathe or dress without help, and his wife had to take over all house-hold chores.

"The pain and fatigue were intense. The muscle injury even had taken my voice away, and it is very difficult for me to swallow food."

Four months after stopping the drug, Lawrence reported, "I have begun to regain some use of my arms and legs, and the muscle pain has receded. The doctor has prescribed a physical fitness program, and I go to the local gym three times a week for an hour of exercises. We continue the fat-free diet, though I have lost too much weight."

Lawrence hopes to be back to normal in another year. He hopes that his voice will have recovered enough that he can return to singing, as he had enjoyed be-ing part of a community group that puts on musical programs for elementary schools and nursing homes.

Recently, Lawrence got his medical records. He discovered that one of the doc-tors who had seen him three years earlier at the famous clinic had thought that his rash might be a drug reaction; he had suggested stopping one or more of Lawrence's medicines to test this theory. Lawrence was deeply disturbed to see this recommendation—because his primary care doctor had not acted on it.

Side effects unrecognized

One study found that when side effects created medical problems that could have been prevented or fixed—but weren't—it was because doctors didn't recognize that the patients' symptoms were in fact side effects.[59]

Dr. Beatrice Golomb at the University of California at San Diego found that when people thought that they were experiencing a drug side effect, scientific evidence strongly suggested that they were typically right. And it was almost always patients—not doctors—who suggested a possible link between a new symptom and a prescribed drug.[60]

Patients were told, "You're just getting old," and "There's nothing wrong with you; it's all in your head."[61] Severe pain was dismissed as "a little discomfort," and doctors implied that their patients were overreacting.[62]

Chillingly, doctors often insisted that patients keep taking medicines causing grave harm—not because they carefully weighed the benefits and risks, but as a result of dismissing the downsides entirely.[64]

Often, as Alesandra found, doctors prescribe additional drugs to manage new symptoms, rather than changing or stopping the drug that is causing them.[65]

> **SAD BUT TRUE**
>
> # 100
>
> Number of pounds a patient must gain as a side effect of a drug before doctors typically consider it a problem worth attention
>
> ❧
>
> Dr. Michael D. Jensen, endocrinologist at the Mayo Clinic, quoted in the *New York Times*[63]

Turning a blind eye

Doctors may get much of their information about drugs from the companies that sell them. The results of this situation are not always ideal. A Harvard Medical School student wondered why his professor so enthusiastically promoted cholesterol drugs "and seemed to belittle a student who asked about side effects."

It turned out that "the professor was not only a full-time member of the Harvard Medical faculty, but a paid consultant to 10 drug companies, including five makers of cholesterol treatments."[66]

Doctors, by the way, believe that patients should view them as the best source of information about drugs.[67] Advertisements reinforce this idea, telling people to "check with your doctor to see if this drug is right for you."

Ties between doctors and manufacturers are common, and concern about them is increasing: "Federal health officials and prosecutors, frustrated that they have been unable to stop illegal kickbacks to doctors from drug and device companies, are investigating doctors who take money for using these products. The move against doctors is part of a diverse campaign to curb industry marketing tactics that enrich doctors but increase health care costs and sometimes endanger patients."[68]

Despite some doctors' enthusiasm for some drugs, troublesome side effects are so common that one group of researchers concluded, "Any symptom in an elderly patient should be considered a drug side effect until proved otherwise."[69]

Their research involved older people, but their conclusion about drugs and side effects is one to keep in mind regardless of the age of the patient.

Side effects unreported

Reports that manufacturers give to the FDA to get approval for a drug typically understate the drug's side effects, for at least three reasons.

First, clinical trials may last just a few months, even if some patients will take the drug for years once it is on the market; trials may not catch side effects that arise over time.

Second, the clinical trial may miss rare side effects; it may include too few people to make it likely that such problems would surface.

Third, the reports are often the *doctors'* interpretation of side effects, not what the patients actually reported. One research study found that doctors routinely say that side effects are less common and less severe than patients report; doctors also omit some reported side effects entirely. As a result, patients who take the drugs in the future can develop problems without being forewarned.[71]

For example, doctors reported that about three out of one hundred patients lost their appetites during treatment for cancer. The patients' own reports showed that more than thirty out of one hundred had this problem. That is, patients had this side effect about ten times as often as doctors said they did.[72]

Relying on the doctors' reports, other physicians may tell their patients, "Almost no one experiences side effects from this treatment. The symptom you're experiencing isn't a side effect."

Once a drug is on the market, doctors are expected to tell the FDA each and every time any patient experiences a serious side effect. This information helps the FDA tell if a drug is more dangerous than originally thought.

SAD BUT TRUE

17-19

Millions of emergency room visits each year due to side effects of medicines

❇

Two unrelated studies, one in the medical journal *BMJ* and one in the *Journal of the American Pharmaceutical Association;* while the studies are dated, the numbers remain plausible[73]

Since doctors routinely deny that new symptoms their patients develop are side effects, it follows that they aren't reporting those side effects to the FDA. These omissions make it even more likely that other doctors will tell patients, "That symptom isn't a side effect of this drug."

Because the FDA doesn't get a complete picture of side effects, it can take them longer than you might expect to recognize problems.

Side effects common

Side effects of drugs are surprisingly common and varied. Consider one side effect: weight gain. The National Institutes of Health noted that some newer drugs "can cause extreme weight gain, worsen cholesterol and lead to diabetes."[74]

The director of the Johns Hopkins Weight Management Center noted that the weight gain ranges from a few pounds to over one hundred pounds and may cause or worsen "diabetes, osteoarthritis, high cholesterol, high blood pressure and other cardiovascular conditions—the very conditions

SAD BUT TRUE

10

Percentage of side effects actually reported by doctors who were required to report 100% of them

❁

Dr. Ethan Basch, reporting in 2010 in the *New England Journal of Medicine* the results of his research involving 467 people with cancer who made 4,034 visits to one of the best cancer centers in the country[78]

for which you might be taking the medication in the first place."[75]

A Mayo Clinic researcher commented, "Many physicians considered a drug's weight gain side effect to be a necessary evil . . . or assumed that only weight gains of 100 pounds or more were worrisome. But drugs that lead people to put on just 10 or 20 pounds a year, if taken for many years, can add up to big problems over time."[76]

Weight gain is a problem only if it's *more than one hundred pounds?* Doctors often say that *losing* just 5-10 percent of one's weight can yield big health gains.[77] For someone weighing 200 pounds, that's 10-20 pounds. Why is *gaining* five to ten times as much unimportant?

Once weight is gained, it is often never lost.[79] In fact, one wonders what portion of the obesity epidemic is a result of prescription drugs, which half the people in this country take daily.[80]

How can people be in charge of their health if they are not told that a drug they've been given is the likely cause of their significant weight gain? How can they decide whether the treatment is delivering more benefits than harm?

Weight gain is just one issue. Another example of unintended downsides of prescription drugs is that people who take high doses of narcotic painkillers after workplace accidents are typically out of work three times as long as people with similar injuries who get smaller doses.[81]

In an article titled, "Be Wary of Narcotics to Treat Back Pain," *Consumer Reports* noted that such drugs often don't help much, and half the people who take them suffer side effects including digestive system and breathing problems. The drugs also result in "a paradoxical increase in pain sensitivity, reduced testosterone levels, and erectile dysfunction. . . . The side effects often outweigh the benefits."[82]

Despite the facts, the volume of such prescriptions is rising—a trend that *Consumer Reports* attributes to extensive marketing.

If you think that you are experiencing side effects, your pharmacist can be very helpful. Pharmacists' whole focus is on the medicines they dispense. They may know more about any given drug than the doctor does and may have a more balanced view of its risks and benefits.

Tracking symptoms

In some cases, tracking your symptoms can help. This approach would not have helped Lawrence, whose problems surfaced years after he started taking the medicine. But it may help some people like Alesandra, whose symptoms show up within a few weeks of starting a new drug.

It helps to keep these records in a spreadsheet or other organized format. (See the two following pages.) Giving your doctor a copy and keeping one yourself can help in three ways. First, you won't forget to mention key points in the rush of the doctor's visit. Second, your doctor can more easily see important patterns. Third, your doctor is likely to take your complaint more seriously. The notes should become part of your medical record, making it less likely that the doctor will simply dismiss your concerns.

Reporting side effects

If you aren't sure that your doctor will report serious side effects, you can report them yourself. (See the box at the end of the chapter). By doing so, you may help other people in the future.

How To Track Your Symptoms

1. **Record each dose of medicine.**
    If you suspect that your symptoms may be related to a drug you are taking, keep a log showing the **date, day of the week**, the **time**, and the **name** and **amount** of each dose of each drug as you take it.

2. **Each time a troublesome symptom arises, record the details.**
    Whether or not you think that a symptom is related to a medicine, it can help to keep a record of your symtom's details, using "**My Symptom Tracker**" (*see next page*) or a document you create that captures similar information:
    a. The **date**, the **day of the week**, and the **time.**
    b. A clear and detailed **description of the symptom**, including **where** it is in your body and **what** it feels like.
    c. **How long** the symptom lasted (*which you can wait to fill in until it has subsided*).
    d. **What you were doing** when the symptom arose (*for example, eating, sleeping, hiking, or sitting at your computer*).
    e. What, if anything, **makes it better** (*such as heat, ice, lying down, or walking*).
    f. What, if anything, **makes it worse.**

My Symptom Tracker

My name _____

Date	Day	Time	Symptom	Where in body	Description	How long	What I was doing	What helped	What made it worse

Figure 1

From *When Health Care Hurts* © 2014 by Elizabeth L. Bewley

How To Find Out About Side Effects and Complications

If you wish to go beyond searches at well-known sites such as the Mayo Clinic, MedlinePlus, WebMD, and Drugs.com, two other options are noted here.

1. **The American Geriatrics Society provides lists of drugs that may cause side effects in older people.** See three documents at http://www.americangeriatrics. org/health_care_professionals/clinical_practice/clinical_ guidelines_recommendations/2012. The first two listed below are found under "Public Education Resources" and the third under "Clinical Tools."
    a. The AGS Beers Criteria **Summary—For Patients & Caregivers**
    b. What to Do and What to Ask Your Healthcare Provider if a Medication You Take is Listed in the "Beers Criteria for **Potentially Inappropriate Medications** to Use in Older Adults"
    c. Beers Criteria—**Pocket Card**

2. **A website run by doctors offers clear comparisons of risks and benefits.** Search **www.thennt.com** to see the percentage of people who benefit from a given treatment compared to the percentage harmed.

How To Report Side Effects to the FDA

1. **Use the MedWatch program.**
   a. **Contact the FDA promptly** at http://www.fda.gov/
      Safety/MedWatch/HowToReport/ucm053074.htm.
   b. The FDA offers options for reporting **online**, by
      phone, and by **mail**.
   c. Find more information on the site under "Your Guide
      to **Reporting Problems to FDA**."
   d. The main phone number is **(800) 332-1088**.

2. **Provide key information:**
   a. How to contact the **patient/person reporting**.
   b. Names of the **doctors/hospital** involved, if any.
   c. The **store** where the drug was purchased.
   d. The **manufacturer**, if known.
   e. The **date** when the product was purchased.
   f. **Product codes** or identifying marks from the prod-
      uct's container.

3. **Follow other steps advised.**
   a. **Keep the product and its container** and labeling.
      (*They provide detailed codes that can help the FDA trace
      the product back to its origin.*)
   b. **Report to the manufacturer and to the store** where
      you purchased the product, if possible, in addition to
      reporting to the FDA. (*The manufacturer's phone num-
      ber may be on the carton or on a leaflet inside.*)

4. **Call a regional FDA Consumer Complaint Coordi-
   nator if you are unsure how to proceed.**
   Phone numbers can be found at http://www.fda.gov/
   Safety/ReportaProblem/ConsumerComplaintCoordina-
   tors/default.htm.

4

"Treatments work for everyone"

Most people think that if the FDA approves a drug or other treatment, it will work for everyone. But many drugs help only a minority of patients, the improvement may be small, and side effects may further reduce the net benefit. Similar issues arise with other treatments, such as surgery.

Efficacy gaps

Rebecca muttered grimly to herself as she stood in the shower. Her job was not going well. She was responsible for some of the financial affairs of a mid-sized multi-national company that was struggling in the tough economy.

By the end of the day, she once again felt defeated. I'm not just running in place, *she thought,* I'm losing ground every day. *She was packing her briefcase when the phone rang.*

She was shocked to hear that her best employee, Kevin, had died of an aneurysm in the airport as he headed for the parking lot. He was 32 years old and left a wife, a two-year-old daughter, and a newborn son.

For Rebecca, it was the last straw. She landed in a psychiatrist's office, diagnosed with depression. The doctor prescribed two drugs, one for depression and one for insomnia. After a series of dose increases, Rebecca reported grogginess, extreme nausea, and faintness. The doctor recommended stomach remedies for the nausea.

SAD BUT TRUE

6

Percentage of people who got better faster when given antibiotics to treat sinus infections—but 12% were harmed by side effects of the drugs

Website run by doctors that bases its conclusions on well-designed scientific studies[83]

Rebecca became confused about basic details of her life. Which shampoo in the shower is mine? What do I normally eat for breakfast?

She also developed a slight tremor. Her employees were eyeing her with concern. After six weeks, she started going home at noon. She could not follow a simple conversation and was sleeping eighteen hours a day.

The doctor stopped prescribing the sleep aid; over time, he upped the dose of the antidepressant to four times the starting level. When she still showed no improvement, he switched her to a second antidepressant and later doubled its dose.

She continued to deteriorate. Her husband said, "The only thing I see happening with this medicine is that you're less engaged with everything. You don't seem engaged with your work at all—you aren't even engaged with roller blading, one of the few things you liked doing. You're more withdrawn, unhappier, more tired, less forthcoming."

That same week, Rebecca was disconcerted to find that random body parts had started to jerk unpredictably. Thoughts of suicide and graphic images of various ways she could kill herself filled her head. With the last bit of fortitude she had, three months into treatment, she called the doctor. He switched her to a third antidepressant. This one worked—or at least it didn't create new problems.

Years later, Rebecca reflected, "Finding the right drug was a brutal process. I almost lost my job. Before I started treatment, no one seemed to know that I was depressed. After I started treatment, everybody at work thought that something was seriously, seriously wrong with me. A few people even thought I was dying."

She continued, "Of course, you're depressed when you start treatment, so every action you have to take feels like climbing a mountain with weights on your back. If I hadn't been obsessive about writing down what was happening, I could easily have committed suicide as a result of the second antidepressant, not realizing that all the suicidal thoughts were a side effect of the drug."

More efficacy gaps

One company boasted that its drug cut pain by at least half in 30 percent of the people taking it.[84] (The other 70 percent didn't fare as well.)

Another drug reduced the number of hot flashes women got from ten a day to four—but women given a placebo (no actual drug) saw a decrease from ten to five or six.[85]

If a doctor says that taking a drug will cut your risk of stroke in half, does that mean that one hundred people at risk will all have strokes if they don't take this drug, but with the medicine only fifty will? Or that untreated, two people out of one hundred at risk will have a stroke, but if all one hundred people take the drug, only one will have a stroke?

Each reflects a 50 percent drop in risk, but the second example is more common with drugs taken to avoid or delay complications of a chronic condition.[87] In fact, analysts discussing a diabetes drug that had sales of $2.6 billion a year pointed out that an almost infinite number of people would have to take the drug for *one person* to see a reduction in complications from diabetes.[88]

Further, when a drug helps people with a severe form of a disease, it may be assumed that people with mild forms will also benefit. But that often is not the case. Results of one study were headlined, "Most People Who Take Blood Pressure Medication Possibly Shouldn't: An independent analysis finds no real benefit for people with mild hypertension."[89]

Drugs are often prescribed even when people aren't in the situation for which they are known to help. For example, a certain drug helps reduce excessive bleeding during surgery; however, about 97 percent of the people given this drug are not in this situation. For them, the drug *reduces* survival rates, causing blood clots leading to heart attacks and strokes.[90]

SAD BUT TRUE

40

Percentage of patients who got a pacemaker implanted when they did not have the condition for which it works

Analysis of five studies involving 5,813 patients, published in the *Archives of Internal Medicine* in 2011 and summarized in the *New York Times,* which reported that 40 percent got "no benefit at all" while experiencing "significant risks" of the surgery itself.[86]

Surgery may also leave patients worse off, in some cases causing permanent disabilities including cognitive decline.[91] Problems can also arise when people who are not good candidates for a procedure are operated on, a common occurrence.

Four results of treatment

Consider two questions when a doctor orders a treatment for you:

- **Does it solve my problem?**
- **Does it create new problems?**

These two questions suggest four possible outcomes. See Figure 2.[93]

The box in the **upper right** is a great place to be: the treatment solves your original problem and doesn't create any others. However, because treatments typically help only about half the time, half the people fall in one of the bottom two boxes.[94]

In the **lower right**, the treatment doesn't help, but it doesn't cause any serious side effects or complications either. That doesn't sound so bad. But if you land in this box, you may waste time and money and just get sicker.

In the **lower left**, the situation is worse. The treatment doesn't help with the original problem, but it creates new ones.

In the **upper left**, the treatment helps but also causes side effects or complications that might be worse than the issue that led you to seek care.

Every person getting any treatment will land in one of these four boxes. It's questionable whether people in the upper left-hand box should continue with the treatment (for example, a drug for a chronic condition). Only people in the upper right-hand box should, almost without question, be encouraged to continue. However, health care professionals too often act as if that box—where only good things happen—is the *only* box.

An individual will get one of four results from a treatment

Images: ©Mary Jackson Dreamstime.com

Helps	Helps, but . . .
	Harms, too
Doesn't help	Doesn't help, and . . .
	Harms, too

Figure 2

In the two upper boxes, the treatment helps with the original problem.
In the two left-hand boxes, side effects/complications cause new harm.

Carrots and sticks

Health care experts often talk about how to get you to take all the drugs prescribed for you, a result they call "compliance" or "adherence."

A national campaign cautions, "If you don't take your medicine as directed, you're putting your health and future at risk." It urges people to "Take the Pledge **Take Your Meds**," (*emphasis in the original*) and offers "I will take my meds" pledge cards.[95]

An insurer wrote, "Taking medicine is an important part of staying healthy. It's very important to take your medicine exactly as ordered."[96]

A doctor wrote in a medical journal that doctors' success depends on "our ability to engage our patients and ensure that they take the medicines we prescribe."[98]

> ### SAD BUT TRUE
>
> # 65
>
> Percentage of metal-on-metal hip implants that went into women and the elderly, when the hip usually works well only in tall, middle-aged men
>
>
>
> *New York Times* article in 2011, based on their analysis, FDA actions, and interviews with a number of orthopedic specialists[97]

A new tool for encouraging compliance is the FICO Medication Adherence Score, which draws on personal information such as age, employment status, and home ownership to predict how likely people are to take their medicine. Doctors, insurance companies, and others will target people with low scores for stepped-up compliance efforts.[99]

These tactics might be fine if all treatments worked for everyone and side effects were no big deal. But neither is the case.

Treatment preferences

Sometimes several good treatments with similar success rates are available, but doctors may use some of the following approaches to try to direct you to choose the option they prefer:

- They imply that you have to decide right now—but unless you're in the emergency room, you usually have days, weeks, or even longer.

- They imply that you don't really have a choice—that the decision is really theirs.
- They tell you about only one solution, or imply that only one solution is good.
- They understate the risks of the option they recommend.

Researchers have found that solutions chosen by doctors often aren't a good fit with the patient's needs, priorities, and values.[100]

By way of analogy, you probably wouldn't let real estate agents choose your next house. While they're the experts, you're the one who knows if you want to live in town or in the country, if you want to have a mansion or a cabin, if you want the master bedroom to be on the ground floor or upstairs, and so forth. You're the one who will be living in the house.

The situation is similar in health care. Doctors may be the experts on the tests and treatments they offer. But you are the expert on your life, and you have a right to choose care that meets your needs. How can you do so, given that you may not know anything about the proposed tests or treatments? See the next two pages for suggestions about questions to ask.

Specific answers are more useful than general ones. For example, it is not very helpful to be told, "This treatment is good for people with bad knees." It is better to know, "This treatment helps two-thirds of athletic men aged 30-40 who have had anterior cruciate ligament tears in the preceding three months."

Ask questions until you feel that you have enough information (to the extent that it exists) to decide if the proposed test or treatment is more likely to *increase* your ability to lead the life you want or to *decrease* it.

SAD BUT TRUE

29

Percentage of people who got metal-on-metal hip implants who had them removed and replaced within six years

New York Times report in 2011 of an analysis by Britain's national health system of all those in Great Britain who got the implants[101]

What To Ask About Tests & Treatments

1. **Four basic questions**
    a. What is this treatment **intended to do**?
    b. **How will we know if it's working** for me?
    c. **When will we know** if it's working for me?
    d. What **big problems** should I watch for, and **what do I do** if they occur?

If a test or treatment is risky, expensive, time-consuming, or otherwise concerning, asking additional questions can help you select ones whose benefits outweigh their risks.

2. **Benefits**
    a. What will this treatment **enable me to do** that I can't do now (*or that I may not be able to do in the future*)?
    b. What do **patients like most** about this treatment?
    c. Will this treatment **solve the problem forever**, or will I need additional treatment now or in the future?

3. **Probability of success**
    a. How is **success defined** for this treatment? (*For example, reduces pain by 25 percent.*)
    b. **How many people out of 100** get that result?
    c. **How am I different** from patients who get good results from this test or treatment (*such as age, gender, height, weight, fitness level, recency of problem's onset, additional health problems and treatments, etc.*)?
    d. Is there **any research** about what happens to patients who have my set of medical conditions, when they get this test or treatment?

4. **Commitment required**
    What else will I have to do to get good results? (*For example, joint surgery is typically not very successful without intensive physical therapy afterwards.*)

What To Ask About Tests & Treatments, cont.

5. **Risks**
   a. What common **side effects or complications** do people experience with this test or treatment?
   b. **How many people out of 100** experience those complications or side effects?
   c. What do **patients dislike most** about this test or treatment?
   d. How much **pain** am I likely to have as a result of this test or treatment, and for how long?
   e. How will this test or treatment **interfere with my ability to lead my normal life**, and for how long? (*For instance, after knee surgery, you might not be able to drive for a number of weeks.*)
   f. How might this test or treatment make any of my **other problems worse**?
   g. What will this treatment **prevent me from doing** that I can do today?

6. **Alternatives**
   What **different tests or treatments** are available for this condition? (*For each of these, all the same questions can be asked.*)

If your doctor cannot provide clear information about risks and benefits, one well-respected resource is **The Cochrane Collaboration**. For non-medical audiences, it offers summaries of its analyses of treatments at http://summaries.cochrane.org.

5

"If you don't get better, it must be your fault"

Doctors and nurses try hard to apply their knowledge and experience to every patient they see. If a patient who they think should be improving instead stays the same or gets worse, the professionals may get frustrated and start taking out their frustration on the patient and family members.

Disrespectful, disruptive, and dangerous

Hannah landed in intensive care on and off for most of the first three months of her life because she just couldn't seem to keep anything down. Her mother, Tiffany, did not produce enough breast milk to meet the baby's needs, so Hannah was fed a combination of breast milk and formula. She vomited up almost everything. They tested her for bacterial infections but didn't find any.

Taking care of her at home was an all-consuming task. Tiffany reported, "I had to clean the feeding tube. I had to draw up her meds. I couldn't turn my back on her. I couldn't leave the room. She was throwing up silently. I would turn around, and she would be choking. I couldn't get sleep."

Eventually, the doctor proposed surgery to tighten the valve between her stomach and her esophagus so that it would be impossible for her to vomit. Then she would retain the formula and start to gain weight.

Tiffany was appalled. Forcing Hannah's body to retain something it clearly didn't want made no sense to her. She heard from parents of other children who'd

SAD BUT TRUE

"Evidence abounds in the form of patient stories regarding demeaning, disrespectful, and dismissive treatment by physicians"

❀

"The Nature and Causes of Disrespectful Behavior by Physicians," written by six doctors and appearing in 2012 in the medical journal *Academic Medicine*[102]

had this surgery, discovering that they still couldn't vomit years later, even if they got a stomach bug and vomiting was the body's natural response.

When she refused the surgery, her relationships with the doctors and nurses became very strained. In their view, she was refusing the ideal treatment for her baby's serious problem. Meanwhile, Hannah continued to lose ground.

Tiffany suspected that Hannah simply was allergic to all the formulas. The doctors scoffed at this idea and criticized her for not knowing the difference between "allergic" and "intolerant." They said, "No baby is intolerant of this formula. This is the one we give babies who can't tolerate anything else."

One rare weekend when Hannah was home from the hospital, Tiffany experimented by giving her only breast milk. Miraculously, Hannah kept down every feeding for two whole days. But on Monday, Tiffany added formula back in, and Hannah started vomiting again.

When she told the doctors about her experiment, Tiffany reported, "I don't know what happened. They refused to hear it. They wouldn't believe it, and it was like I was talking to a wall."

Another woman with a baby in intensive care offered Tiffany some of her extra breast milk for Hannah. Two medical professionals supported the idea, but told Tiffany very emphatically that she had to keep it a secret, especially from the baby's main doctor. Tiffany agreed, but didn't understand why it was such an issue.

Before long, the doctor did find out and was very angry. He gave orders forbidding Tiffany from feeding her daughter. Despite those orders, a nurse wrote a negative comment in Hannah's chart criticizing Tiffany for not feeding her baby.

Then Tiffany found out that using informally donated breast milk was against hospital policy, for good reason. Breast milk can contain residues of medicines the mother is taking and other harmful substances.

Once she understood the issues, she researched other options. She discovered that there are human milk banks, just as there are blood banks. They screen donated breast milk, pasteurize it to eliminate bacteria, and blend it to get standardized calorie counts, ranging from 13 to 30 calories per ounce. But Hannah's doctor claimed, in error, that breast milk contained only 21 calories per ounce, while Hannah needed 24 calories. He refused to listen to any of Tiffany's explanations.

When she persisted, he said, "How are you going to pay for it? Banked milk is too expensive. Your insurance won't cover it. You don't have enough money, so this isn't even an option."

Tiffany figured that she would worry about the money later, but he refused to write the prescription.

Tiffany's questions typically went unanswered. For example, she asked why a replacement feeding tube was inserted three times as far into Hannah's tiny belly as the previous one had been. Her question was ignored.

SAD BUT TRUE

1 in 9

Doctors who said they see other doctors engage in disruptive behavior that can harm patients every day

❦

Study of more than 840 doctors reported in a white paper sponsored by the American College of Physician Executives in 2011[103]

Hannah stopped vomiting, but she was very irritable. Ten days later, an X-ray showed that the feeding tube had been inserted so far that it went right past her stomach. No one even apologized for this life-threatening mistake.

When a replacement tube was inserted correctly, Hannah promptly started vomiting again, a fact omitted from her medical records. Tiffany asked that the digestive system specialist (gastroenterologist) be called about Hannah's feeding program. She was told that he had approved it. Much later, she found out that he had not even been consulted and was very upset when he found out what had happened.

Tiffany noted, "Because I didn't know my rights, I didn't know how to act. They were always making me feel like I didn't have a right to this or a right to that, or I shouldn't be acting this way or doing that."

While Hannah was in the hospital, social workers repeatedly showed up, peppering Tiffany with questions about her family, home, income, and so forth. They wrote into Hannah's records that Tiffany was severely depressed. She felt under attack on all fronts, concluding that they used her depression as an excuse to further discount anything she might say.

One day, she asked if she could take Hannah outside for a few minutes to walk

SAD BUT TRUE

26

Percentage of doctors who admit that they themselves have engaged in disruptive behavior

🪷

Study of more than 840 doctors reported in a white paper sponsored by the American College of Physician Executives in 2011[104]

on the grass under the trees. The nurses refused and wrote in Hannah's chart that Tiffany had tried to run away from the hospital with the baby.

Tiffany was told that she was the reason that Hannah was failing to thrive. The next time Hannah was discharged, Tiffany found a phone message waiting when she carried the baby into the house. The hospital had reported her for child endangerment, and a social worker needed to visit to decide whether Hannah—and Tiffany's other three children—were safe. Tiffany was mortified and angry.

The social worker was very impressed by what she saw at the house, including the very careful records Tiffany kept of Hannah's complicated medication schedule, feedings, and other care.

She told Tiffany that the hospital was out of line for reporting her, because there was not a shred of evidence that Tiffany was anything other than an organized, careful, loving mother. She offered to testify in court.

Tiffany was exhausted and coping with some other undiagnosed medical problems of her own. She was also managing Hannah's hospitalizations by herself; her husband was busy taking care of their other young children.

Having to justify herself to the social worker was the last straw. Tiffany decided to take Hannah to a different hospital, further away from home. There, doctors quickly detected that Hannah could not tolerate corn, the common ingredient in all the formulas she had been given. They immediately prescribed banked human milk, and the baby began a long, slow recovery from the abusive effects of constantly being fed food that made her violently ill.

Hannah's need for human milk was not an oddity. Two years later, a children's hospital in another part of the country reported that it feeds only breast milk to newborns in intensive care, because "the evidence is overwhelming" that it's best for the vulnerable infants.[105] And insurance typically covers the cost.

Besides providing care that nearly killed her baby, the doctors and hospital staff engaged in what Tiffany termed "psychological warfare," repeatedly criticizing, discounting, and belittling her. No matter what action or response she chose, she was "wrong." In short, instead of saying, "Hannah has a problem that we haven't been able to diagnose," they said, in effect, "You are a bad mother."

Erroneous assumptions and disrespect

Doctors and nurses may assume that the diagnoses you're given are correct, that treatments work for everyone, that side effects are no big deal, and that we have the best health care in the world.

Therefore, if you continue to deteriorate, they may start looking outside the realm of health care for an explanation.

They may start to wonder if you are the problem. Maybe you aren't really following the treatment plan. Maybe you are deliberately sabotaging your care. Maybe you just don't want to get better. These suspicions may lead them to start treating you (or family members) as if you are the enemy.

Sometimes patients' experiences with doctors and nurses remind me of American Indians' experiences with Europeans. The Indians never had a chance. The Europeans were certain of their own superiority and sought to impose their perspective on the Indians. Patients, too, are often treated as inferior beings whose role is simply to be subdued into compliance.

Watch for these red flags:

- Doctors or nurses deny basic facts about the patient's condition that are obvious to casual observers.
- Doctors or nurses ignore serious issues that the patient or family member raises or brush them off without any plausible explanation.
- Doctors or nurses blame the patient or family member for the patient's failure to improve—when no facts support this stance.

How To Address Red Flags

1. **Learn your rights.**
   If the hospital has a statement of patient rights (*which may be titled "Patient Rights and Responsibilities"*), read it carefully and keep a copy.

2. **Find out how to contact Patient Relations.**
   This hospital department may also be known as the Patient Ombudsman or Patient Advocate. Be sure to learn what to do if you need help when they are not available.

3. **Get help from an advocate.**
   Choose someone you trust who can help you sort through all the information and be a sounding board to help you make good decisions.

6

"Doctors focus on the important stuff"

Doctors may undergo training for a dozen years or even more, between premed in college, medical school, residency, and specialized training after that. It only makes sense that they would focus on major, complex issues and not waste their time on the little stuff. But what if it's the little stuff that makes the critical difference in the patient's recovery?

A lack of focus on details in the hospital

Don was 65 when he was diagnosed with leukemia and treated with daily injections of a drug to slow the cancer's progression. After a few months, when he developed a fever and muscle pains, he was admitted to the hospital. Within days, he had become so weak that he was unable even to lift his head off the pillow.

Many years later Elaine remembered her frustration with Don's doctors. She kept saying that the cancer drug must be the culprit, but the doctors kept testing Don for obscure and unlikely diseases. When they couldn't figure out his problem, they told Elaine that he was going to die. She felt that he wasn't getting the right attention, but didn't know what to do. He was in a prestigious hospital with a reputation for excellent care.

One day about a month after he was admitted, Elaine reported, "All of a sudden he was scooped up and taken to a gorgeous suite. It was just palatial. He was given everything, all by himself."

Now Elaine could stay when Don was being treated.

"I peeked through the curtain one day while they were turning him, and I saw a bedsore on his lower back. It was four inches long, and I could see down to his bone. Then I find out that he's got them all over. He had four of them."

Neither Don nor Elaine had been told that Don had bedsores, also known as pressure ulcers or decubitus ulcers. His were all Stage IV, meaning that the tissue from the skin down to the bone had been injured or destroyed.

Bedsores develop because of unrelieved pressure on bony parts of the body when an individual stays in one position for hours at a time, as Don did because he was too weak to move.

They also arise from friction or shear when patients slip out of position or drag themselves in bed—or are dragged by caregivers—instead of being lifted.

Bedsores can start to develop in as little as two hours. Drew Griffin, a certified wound care nurse with eighteen years of experience, observed that they arise even faster if the patient is at high risk due to factors including immobility, other medical problems, poor nutrition, and dehydration.[108]

Kate Suchmann, Professor of Nursing at Vermont Technical College, noted, "The biggest risk for bedsores besides pressure is poor nutrition. And people don't want to drink enough fluids. Fluids are essential for tissue function. So patients need to move, drink, eat."[109] But in the entire month that Don had been there, no one had said anything at all to Don or Elaine about preventing or treating bedsores. And Don continued to deteriorate.

After he had been in the hospital for nearly three months, Elaine's theory about his underlying illness was proven correct. Doctors concluded that Don had drug-induced lupus, a rare but known side effect of the cancer medicine he was getting. Soon after they changed his treatment, he was well enough to be moved to a rehabilitation facility. A month later, he was sent home.

However, he still had four Stage IV bedsores. The Mayo Clinic notes that even Stage I and Stage II pressure ulcers can take months to heal. Those in Stage III and Stage IV "are more difficult to treat."[110]

As Elaine pointed out, "The skin may grow over it, but you're missing the muscles and tendons and nerves. All that tissue that was destroyed and had to be removed because it was dead never comes back."

For six months, nurses came twice a day, seven days a week, to change Don's bandages and clean the wounds. Then one of the registered nurses, Kate Suchmann, who later went on to teach, trained Elaine to do much of this critical, painstaking work.

Suchmann said, "Elaine is very probably the only reason he's alive. She is very gifted, focused, and precise—and she was always asking questions."[112]

SAD BUT TRUE

100

Percentage of bedsores deemed preventable

Medicare, which terms bedsores "never" events, meaning that they are preventable and therefore should never occur[111]

For years, Don's and Elaine's lives revolved around dealing with his bedsores. More than 10 years later, Don said, "I have tremendous pain," and Elaine rattled off a list of medicines he was taking to treat the pain and nerve damage.

Medicare, the federal health insurance program for the elderly and disabled, typically won't even pay hospitals to treat severe bedsores like Don's, because they should have prevented them from developing.[113]

Don didn't have bedsores when he arrived at the hospital. Then doctors focused on complex diagnostic tests and other sophisticated activities. Inadequate focus was put on the basic—but essential—tasks that nurses often perform, such as repositioning patients frequently to prevent bedsores. More than a decade later, Don continues to pay the price.

Is the problem that there isn't enough time or technology or money or staff? No, it is what Dr. Don Berwick, a leader in efforts to improve the results that patients get from health care, described as "a deficiency of will and ambition," a failure by hospital executives to focus on delivering better care to patients.[114]

See the box on the next page for action steps to take to prevent bedsores.

How To Prevent Bedsores

1. **Learn about the risk.**
   a. Go to **bradenscale**.com.
   b. Click on Products>Braden Scale for Predicting Pressure Sore Risk. This **one-page quiz** is widely used to estimate the likelihood that a specific patient will develop bedsores.

2. **Create a plan** with the doctor, addressing key questions:
   a. Is this **patient at risk** for pressure ulcers?
   b. **What will you do** to prevent pressure ulcers from developing?
   c. What will the **nurses** do?
   d. What can the **patient** do?
   e. What can **family members** do?

3. **Follow up.**
   a. Confirm that **planned actions take place**.
   b. Ask to see the results of **assessments of the patient's skin**.
   c. Ask for an **assessment by a dietitian** if the patient doesn't eat or drink much.

A lack of guidance on details of care at home

It was the first nice Saturday in weeks, and I had set off early in the morning on my bicycle. My bike bag held maps of seven counties and four bottles of water. I promised my husband only that I would be home in time for dinner.

After I had ridden ten or fifteen miles, I ended up at the top of a hill posted with signs saying, "15 percent grade." I didn't know what they meant. The road was curved, so I couldn't see more than fifty feet ahead. Very soon, I was startled to realize that I was going faster than I'd ever ridden before. Much, much faster.

I gently squeezed the brakes, but hit a patch of gravel as I came upon a sharp curve much too fast. The bike wobbled, and for a second I was suspended in a cocoon of disbelief. Then I hit the ground. I bounced and rolled, bounced and rolled, and bounced and rolled again. Later, the policeman who responded to a bystander's 911 call looked at the computer on my bicycle and told me that I'd been going 44 miles per hour when I crashed.

After my husband arrived in the emergency room, a nurse told him, "If your wife hadn't been wearing a bicycle helmet, you wouldn't be standing here talking to her. You'd be making funeral arrangements."

Six hours later, I got the tally of my injuries: broken right wrist; left arm flayed raw from elbow to hand; puncture wounds from pieces of gravel half an inch in diameter, embedded so far that no one noticed them for the first five hours; massive hematoma on my left hip, meaning that a blood vessel broke and bled into the surrounding tissue, making it look as if I'd attached half a honeydew melon to my side; and extensive abrasions—road rash—on my right thigh and both knees.

Given all these injuries, what caused me the most pain and greatest subsequent trauma? The gauze pads they prescribed in the emergency room to cover my entire left forearm, which had lost layers of skin to the asphalt.

They told my husband to change the many gauze pads twice a day to avoid infection. The first time he tried, every bit of healing tissue stuck to the gauze and tore off my arm as each bandage in turn was removed, causing extensive bleeding and oozing and excruciating pain.

The next day, as my husband tried to complete this hour-long task, he said, "We have to stop. You've gone chalk white. You're going to pass out." We called the doctor, asking for an appointment to get the bandage changed and also explaining that my arm felt more painful, swollen, and hot than it had before.

The doctor's office refused to give me an appointment, saying dismissively, "We don't change dressings." We begged and pleaded. After several phone calls, a clearly irritated staff member grudgingly agreed that we would come in.

The first thing the doctor and nurse did when they entered the examining room was to rebuke me, again, for insisting on an office visit. Then they pulled off the gauze, again tearing off all the new tissue and again causing excruciating pain. As they were preparing to re-bandage my arm, a senior physician came in to inspect it. He pointed out to the less-experienced doctor that my arm was infected and prescribed antibiotics.

He had turned to leave when I again blurted out that ripping off the healing tissue twice a day couldn't be good. He looked at me quizzically and said, "If the gauze is sticking, use Teflon-coated gauze pads. They won't stick."

"WHAT?!" my husband and I both exclaimed. "Where do you get them? What are they called?"

He told us, we got some, and the horrible, hour-long, twice-daily trauma was over. All it really took was a few words. You would think it would be automatic to give emergency room patients who leave with wound dressings clear instructions for how to change the bandages and how to handle common problems— such as skin sticking to the gauze. But we hadn't been given this information.

Don's bedsores were far more serious than my bicycling injuries. Yet even in my simpler situation, the lack of focus on small details led to unnecessary pain, a serious infection, and the need for extra office visits, antibiotics, and painkillers.

Why hadn't they spoken up sooner? It is standard in health care to focus on the high-tech, high-skill activities that the *doctor* handles. Changing bandages is a low-tech activity that *we* were to handle. Consequently, it was not given focused attention—despite its very critical role in healing.

See the box on the next page for suggestions about how to handle unfamiliar care tasks at home.

How To Manage Care at Home

1. **Ask questions to help you plan and prepare.**
   a. **What is the task**?
   b. When is the **first time** I should do it? (*The day you leave the hospital? The next day?*)
   c. **How often** am I to do it?
   d. **How many people** will it take in my case?
   e. **What equipment or supplies** do I need?
   f. **Where** can I get them?
   g. **What steps** are involved? (*You may need to rephrase the question: "I assume that the first step is to wash my hands. The second is to lay out the supplies. Then what?"*)
   h. Can you give me **written instructions** to refer to?

2. **Ask about trouble spots.**
   a. If untrained aides were handling this task, what kinds of **problems** might arise? (*For example, if the task is changing bandages, what signs or symptoms would suggest that the wound is infected? If the task is changing an oxygen tank, how would I know if oxygen weren't actually reaching the patient?*)
   b. What **steps** should I take **to solve** those problems?

3. **Find out how and when to get help.**
   a. When would I **need to get professional help**?
   b. Who and **what number** do I call? Does the answer change if it is a night or weekend?

7

"The diagnosis you get is correct"

Misdiagnosis is surprisingly common, as is the harm it can cause. At a minimum, being treated for a disease you don't have is unlikely to help you. Sources of diagnostic errors range from discounting patients' genuine, significant symptoms to grossly misinterpreting test results.

Five diagnostic errors

In the first four cases described in this chapter, doctors dismissed the possibility that their patients might have physical problems that needed prompt medical attention. In the fifth case, the doctor relied on test results that his own orders rendered invalid.

Below are flawed conclusions that doctors drew:

1. An individual had deliberately interfered with the testing.
2. A graduate student lied about her symptoms.
3. A child was just seeking attention.
4. A college student had a problem that was all in her head.
5. An emergency room patient had a common condition and did not need emergency care.

Ignoring test results

Discovery Health Channel's program Mystery Diagnosis *profiled a woman with severe breathing problems.*

During a visit to a lung specialist, she was asked to blow hard into a tube attached to a machine that measures airflow into and out of the lungs.

She did so poorly that the doctor rebuked her for not trying hard enough, did not examine her further, and then referred her for psychiatric counseling for her "bad attitude."

Months later, after she had seen many doctors and continued to deteriorate, a new doctor decided to take x-rays. She found a large tumor that filled most of one lung. It was no surprise that the patient had done badly on the breathing test.[116]

In this case, even though the test the doctor performed gave completely accurate results, the doctor refused to even consider the possibility that the test might be right. Instead of ordering another test to try to confirm or disprove the results of the first one, the doctor simply assumed that the patient wasn't cooperating.

Dismissing reported symptoms as impossible

In December of my second year of graduate school, I came down with an earache. I went to the student health center, but after a dozen visits and assorted drug therapies, my ear was still full of fluid and I still couldn't hear right. After five months, the doctor sliced my eardrum open to drain the fluid. Then he told me that my problems were over: he had suctioned out all the liquid and no more would accumulate.

I slept badly that night. I kept waking up every half-hour or so, each time because the pillow had a new wet spot on it. The cotton ball in my ear had become saturated, and fluid had overflowed onto the pillow. In the dark, I groggily removed the soggy cotton ball, threw it on a mat beside my bed, and inserted a dry one. In the morning, there were 13 discarded cotton balls on the mat.

After a few days, the fluid slowed and then stopped; the slit in the eardrum had closed. I saw the surgeon a couple days later. I told him about the 13 soggy cotton balls and the continuous leak of fluid over the weekend.

"Oh, that's ridiculous!" he snapped. "That didn't happen!"

I was stunned into silence. He told me that I was cured and ended the appointment.

My ear once again full of fluid, I returned a week later, taking his first available appointment.

He decided to schedule a procedure for a month later to slice my eardrum open—again—but this time he was going to put in a drainage tube. On the appointed day, he suctioned out my ear, but couldn't get the tube to stay in.

> **SAD BUT TRUE**
>
> # 12
>
> Millions of preventable misdiagnoses given to non-hospitalized patients each year; half have the potential to cause severe harm
>
>
>
> Researchers writing in 2014 in the journal *BMJ Quality & Safety*[17]

He stepped away to prepare for another try. When he returned, he stopped short, incredulous. He exclaimed, "There's more fluid in your ear!"

It turned out that cerebrospinal fluid was leaking from my brain into my ear. It was going first through a small hole in the membrane surrounding my brain, just above my ear, and then through a larger hole in the roof of my middle ear. Plans were quickly made for me to have brain surgery.

It's not surprising that the doctor didn't figure out what was wrong for five months. My situation was very unusual. But when I told him about the 13 soggy cotton balls in April, he rejected the facts because they didn't fit his assumptions.

Acting as if the doctor's theory *trumps the patient's reality is very dangerous*. If he'd succeeded in placing the tube in my ear, he would have forced open a direct and quasi-permanent channel from the outside air to the inside of my brain. Potentially fatal bacterial meningitis could easily have followed.

Because the doctor denied that my symptoms were possible, I didn't get the life-saving brain surgery I needed until five or six weeks after it first became crystal clear that something was seriously wrong. In one realm in my life, I was on the dean's list in a competitive graduate school. In another realm, I was treated as if I could not be trusted to convey the simplest of facts.

SAD BUT TRUE

40,000
to
80,000

Number of deaths each year due to "delayed, missed, [or] incorrect diagnoses"

Study published in 2012 in *JAMA (Journal of the American Medical Association)*[118]

Dismissing a patient's report as attention-seeking

A book called Wall of Silence *tells the story of an eight-year-old girl, Elizabeth (no relation to the author), who had been treated for kidney cancer. When she told her parents that the cancer had returned, her doctors refused to examine her. They said that she was only seeking attention.*

Over three months, the child lost a third of her body weight. Her mother called the doctors nearly two dozen times. Never examining their patient, they continued to tell her mother to ignore her attention-seeking behavior.

When she became almost entirely non-responsive, her doctors committed her to a psychiatric ward. After she had a seizure, they ordered an MRI, which showed that the cancer had long since spread to her spine and brain.

Grueling treatment over the next year saved her life. However, the delay of many months caused by her doctors' unwarranted assumption that her problem was psychological left her permanently paralyzed from the waist down.[119]

One key point stands out: her doctors were swift to label her emotionally disturbed when she implied that she knew what was happening in her own body. Think about that for a moment.

Believing that a physical disorder is caused by a mental one

Stacy squirmed uncomfortably in her seat. She looked at her watch. The hour-long class had another seven minutes to go. Could she make it? She tried to distract herself by focusing fiercely on the professor's words and writing down as much as she could of what he was saying. Then she started quietly gathering her belongings, anticipating the end of the class. Finally, finally, the bell rang. She grabbed her bag and almost jogged to the restroom.

It was a few months into her sophomore year in college, and she had recently started having trouble sitting through classes without a bathroom break. Two of her classes were 90 minutes, and one was two hours. And now she couldn't even make it through the shortest one, 60 minutes.

As soon as the problem had arisen, she had gone to the doctor she had been seeing for years. He told her that the problem was psychosomatic—all in her head. She was a straight-A student and was used to accomplishing anything she set out to do.

"I must be going crazy!" she scolded herself. "How can I not stop this—especially because I know it's psychosomatic? This is really insane that I can't seem to stop!"

SAD BUT TRUE

1/3

Proportion of people found by autopsies to have been misdiagnosed who probably would have lived had they been treated for the disease they actually had

Dr. Atul Gawande, in his book *Complications*[120]

Five years later, she said, "It was unbearable for me, because it does ruin your life if you have to go to the bathroom all the time." She continued to suffer month after month.

She reported, "When I had finals that would be an hour to two hours long, it was especially hard. I had to go to the professor in advance and explain that I couldn't make it through the exam. Usually what they would do was send a TA [teaching assistant] into the bathroom with me." She found this arrangement very humiliating. But the professors wanted to make sure that she wasn't cheating, using bathroom breaks to check her notes.

After a year with no improvement—but with more symptoms such as stomach pain—Stacy agreed to see her parents' doctor. He examined her briefly and then asked, "What do you drink?" Stacy thought it an odd question, but explained that she had gotten in the habit of drinking large quantities of diet cola—there was a soda machine around every corner on the college campus, and the caffeine helped her to stay alert.

The doctor told her very emphatically to cut out the soda completely. He explained that its caffeine, carbonation, and acid could irritate her bladder and account for all her symptoms, including abdominal pain. Ten days later, all her symptoms were gone; they never returned.

SAD BUT TRUE

96

Percentage of doctors who say that diagnostic errors could "sometimes" or "always" be prevented; sadly, misdiagnosis nevertheless remains very common

Survey of more than 6,400 doctors in 2011[121]

Several years later, Stacy still found the experience disturbing: "I suffered for a year because I thought it was all in my head."

It's worth noting that the problem Stacy experienced wasn't due to a germ or a structural abnormality—the kinds of things that can show up on physical exams or on lab tests. Her doctor could have run a dozen tests and come up with nothing, reinforcing his belief that the symptoms were all in her head.

Doctors sometimes assume that a patient with puzzling symptoms is mentally ill. Psychiatric illnesses are important and should be appropriately treated. But telling you that you have an unspecified mental illness when what they really mean is, "I haven't figured out what's wrong with you," is enough to *drive* the most stalwart person insane.

Ignoring ways in which test results can be misleading

Amber, age 26, lay in the emergency room. She couldn't move her arms, her mind repeatedly blanked out for several minutes at a time, her vision was blurred, and she was extremely dizzy. Her stomach hurt so much that she hadn't had anything to eat or drink for many hours.

The doctor said, "I think you're just dehydrated."

They put an IV line in her arm and attached a bag of dextrose solution to drip into her vein. Shortly after the bag of sugar water had emptied, a technician showed up to draw blood. He explained, "The doctor wants to see if you have diabetes."

Amber said, "That's going to read high in sugar from the IV bag of dextrose I just got."

The technician replied, "It's OK. I'm drawing blood from your other arm." Amber's mother objected to this view, pointing out that blood travels throughout the body, but the technician just shrugged and finished drawing Amber's blood.

Later, the doctor came and said, "Your blood sugar level is high. I think you're diabetic." He sent her home with a glucose test meter and test strips, telling her to test her blood sugar level regularly.

When she was discharged, Amber was still having trouble controlling her arms and legs. She was still having trouble holding a conversation, and her mind continued to blank out. She reported, "I spent the next week in bed in severe pain, unable to function."

Amber's primary care doctor later confirmed what Amber already knew: she did not have diabetes. Instead, she had a potentially life-threatening brain infection that the emergency room doctor failed to diagnose.

SAD BUT TRUE

75+

Number of years that rates of major misdiagnoses discovered during autopsies have stayed the same

Dr. Atul Gawande, in his book *Complications*, discussing research going back to 1938[122]

What went wrong with her medical test? After all, the correct patient was tested, and the test done was the one the doctor ordered. The lab work was accurate. The results were recorded under the correct patient's name. The doctor who ordered the test received the results and read them.

However, the test led to a completely incorrect conclusion, a result easily predicted even by a patient who was mentally challenged at the time.

Perhaps the doctor simply ordered the blood test and read the results without thinking about the dextrose drip. Or he may have ordered the blood test before the IV line went in, but the busy lab just didn't get to Amber until after she had had roughly a quart of sugar water infused into her veins. The problem is that the professionals didn't connect the dots.

Preventing diagnostic errors

The popular television show *House* features the curmudgeonly, often hostile—but brilliant—Dr. Gregory House who can come up with an accurate diagnosis when others can't.

He is permanently pain-wracked because of a disability resulting from a misdiagnosis, perhaps providing the inspiration for him to work to spare others a similar fate.

The premise of the show—that doctors sometimes don't recognize the patient's malady—is based in fact. That said, tools are available to improve diagnostic accuracy.

One of these is a computer program named Isabel, sort of an electronic version of Dr. House—minus the limp and the attitude.

The program was created by a father whose three-year-old daughter Isabel nearly died as a result of misdiagnosis. One study showed that using Isabel resulted in important changes in diagnosis 14 percent of the time.[124]

But such tools are rarely used, and initiatives to improve diagnostic accuracy are rare. As one writer commented, "Under the current medical system, doctors, nurses, lab technicians and hospital executives are not actually paid to come up with the right diagnosis. They are paid to perform tests and to do surgery and to dispense drugs."[125]

Misunderstanding accuracy rates

Many doctors assume that a single diagnostic test is all that's needed to tell if you have a particular disease. But tests are often less reliable than you—and your doctor—might believe. According to Michael Blastland and Andrew Dilnot in their book *The Numbers Game*, only about 8 percent of doctors did the math right when asked to calculate how likely it was that a person whose test results indicated that they had a disease actually had it. The rest of them, they said, were "hopelessly confused."[126]

Consider an example.

Assume that only 10 people out of 1000 screened for a condition like diabetes actually have the disease. The other 990 people are fine. Assume that the test is 90 percent accurate. These numbers mean that 10 percent of the 990 people who are fine will be told that they are sick. These erroneous results are called false positives, and in this case they snag 99 people.

In this example, the test is also 90% accurate for the 10 people who have diabetes. As a result, the reports will indicate that 9 of them have diabetes, and will mistakenly note that the 10th person doesn't, an error called a false negative.

In total, 9 people who have diabetes and 99 who don't—a total of 108 people—will all be told that they have the disease when only 8 percent of the 108 actually do.

Most doctors incorrectly assumed that 90 percent of the people who tested positive do have the disease. False positives, if left unchallenged, can lead to unnecessary treatment.

Patients who test positive (on tests with an accuracy profile similar to the one in the example) can be told, "This test came back positive,

SAD BUT TRUE

92

Percentage of doctors who gave very wrong answers when given facts about a test's accuracy and asked to say what the odds were that someone who tested positive for cancer actually had the disease

❀

The Numbers Game by Michael Blastland and Andrew Dilnot reporting on research involving 24 doctors[127]

but 92% of the people who test positive don't actually have the disease. We need to run a second, different test. The odds that both tests will give incorrect answers are very small."

Other mistakes in testing occur in one out of thirty office visits.[128] The doctor may order the wrong test; the lab may perform the test incorrectly; or the lab might even perform the wrong test entirely. Thus, the results can be meaningless, even without considering the issue of false positives and false negatives.

The boxes on the next two pages explain how to get more meaningful results from medical tests and how to increase the odds that the diagnosis you get will be accurate.

How To Get Useful Results from Tests

1. **Prepare.**
   a. Ask what might **skew** the results. (*For example, eating a high-fat food such as cheesecake shortly before having a cholesterol test might distort the results.*)
   b. Read **pretest instructions** as soon as you get them; follow them carefully.

2. **Track.**
   a. Write down the **name of the test** and what it is for.
   b. Ask **when you will get the results**, how (*phone, mail, and so forth*), and from whom.
   c. Ask to be sent a copy of the **actual test results**, not just a message or postcard saying, "Your test was fine."
   d. **Note on your calendar** the date by which you should receive the results (*or two dates, if you expect a call followed by a paper or electronic report*).
   e. **Call** the doctor's office promptly if you don't get the results when expected.

3. **Follow up.**
   a. Check to see that the **results correctly report** your name and birth date and the name of the test. (*Doctors' offices sometimes mix up test results.*)
   b. If a test shows that you have a problem, ask how this **conclusion can be confirmed**. Often a different test can be run, to help address false positives and other errors.

How To Get a More Accurate Diagnosis

1. **Track your symptoms** (see Chapter 3).

2. **If no diagnosis is made, give more information:**
    a. **Medicines/recreational drugs/vitamins** you take.
    b. **Alcohol** and **tobacco** use.
    c. **Food** and **beverages** you normally eat and drink.
    d. **New detergents** or **cosmetics** recently started.
    e. **Time use** (*activities you spend the most time on, such as driving a delivery truck, playing video games, teaching first grade, and so forth*).
    f. The **physical environment** you're typically in.
    g. **Exercise habits** and **sleep patterns**.

3. **If a diagnosis doesn't ring true:**
    a. Use the **Mayo Clinic Symptom Checker** at http://www.mayoclinic.org/symptom-checker/select-symptom/itt-20009075 to help identify other conditions that have symptoms like yours.
    b. Ask why other conditions that fit were **ruled out**.
    c. Ask if any of your **symptoms don't fit** the diagnosis.
    d. Ask if you might have **more than one problem**.[129]

4. **If you doubt a diagnosis of mental illness:**
    a. Ask **what additional symptoms** would be expected.
    b. If such indicators **don't apply to you**, point that out.

5. **If several treatments have not helped:**
    a. **Document each treatment**: dates started and ended and any changes in symptoms that seemed to result.
    b. Show your doctor the list and ask if it might be time to **revisit the diagnosis**.

6. **If you don't feel heard:**
    a. Get a **second opinion**.
    b. If necessary, get a **new doctor**.

8

"You don't need to know what's going on"

It's common in health care to assume that the professionals have everything under control and that patients don't need much information. But you need to know what's going on as events unfold, for at least three reasons. First, feedback you provide when you hear the plan can result in important changes to your care. Second, your anxiety level can be dramatically reduced if you know what to expect. Third, you may be the one who needs to take the next steps, which is hard to do if you don't know what they are.

Asking the reasons for instructions you are given

Michelle fell off a ladder while fixing some Christmas lights that had come loose outside her suburban Virginia home. She landed awkwardly on her leg, and the pain was intense.

She called her doctor, but it was December 23 and his office had closed at noon for the holiday. He instructed her to go to an urgent care clinic, where they took x-rays and sent her home. Two minutes after her doctor's office reopened on December 26, she got an urgent call from him: her leg was badly broken, and she needed emergency surgery.

At the hospital, Michelle refused to let the first available surgeon operate on her. She had previously had a bad experience with an unfamiliar surgeon and was taking no chances. She ended up parked on a gurney (a stretcher) in a hall-

SAD BUT TRUE

90

Percentage of patients in the hospital who didn't know what doctor was in charge of their care

❧

Study of 2,807 patients summarized in the *Archives of Internal Medicine*[130]

way in the emergency room for almost ten hours while she waited for a surgeon she knew and trusted to see her.

Five or six hours after Michelle arrived, a nurse flipped back the sheet to uncover Michelle's right leg. She handed Michelle an uncapped marker and said, "Sign your name on your leg."

Cautious about blindly following orders, Michelle asked, "Why?"

The nurse said impatiently, "It's so the surgeon will know which leg to operate on."

Michelle blanched. "But my left leg is the one that's broken!"

The nurse did not look at Michelle's legs at all. She looked at her chart.

"Oh, so it is," she said.

Then she uncovered the correct leg.

"Sign your name."

Michelle was stupefied. The nurse did not even apologize.

Michelle's experience highlights two key points about mistakes in hospitals. First, measures such as requiring patient signatures on body parts may have been put in place to prevent errors.

Second, health care workers can defeat the safety features if they take shortcuts. Telling Michelle to sign her name on her leg without explaining why could have created a huge problem. The nurse seemed to be going through the motions without honoring the intent of the safeguard.

One industry insider observed, "Health care systems have always transferred uncertainty and risk to the patient. Managers, doctors and nurses are in control; they have certainty, it is the patient who usually does not know what is going to happen, or when or why. The risk is taken by the patient rather than the doctor."[131]

Ironically, informed consent forms are typically not written to inform consent. Would you immediately realize that a "percutaneous endoscopic gastrostomy tube" is a feeding tube?[132]

Attempts to simplify the language are resisted, because informed consent forms are viewed as "legal tools." That is, they aren't intended to help you understand medical actions that could radically change or end your life. They are intended to make it harder for you to sue.[133]

Doctors and nurses often resist allowing patients and family members to act as part of the care team.

In one case, a hospital set up a rapid response system. Patients or family members could call for help if the patient was crashing and wasn't getting needed attention. Professionals derided this plan, saying that it would lead to "calls to pick up dirty linens." That is, patients and family members were assumed to be so incompetent that they wouldn't be able to tell the difference between dying and housekeeping.

What actually happened? In every case when family members called for help, the rapid response team ended up rushing the patient to intensive care.[135]

Poor communication between patients and doctors "can increase risk for injury or death. . . . 'More serious adverse events are caused by communication problems than any other thing.'"[136] Keeping patients and family members out of the loop is dangerous for the patient.

> SAD BUT TRUE
>
> # 55
>
> Percentage of patients in the hospital whose reports of the diagnoses they had been given were different from the diagnoses shown in their charts
>
> ✿
>
> Study of 233 patients published by the Mayo Clinic in 2010[134]

Refusing unexpected tests

Tom, age 45, was in the hospital receiving IV antibiotics to treat an abdominal infection, and he was feeling much better. The extreme pain that he'd had in his belly was completely gone, but he knew that he had to keep getting the antibiotics for a while longer. He looked up when an orderly entered the room, pushing a wheelchair.

"Okay, buddy," the orderly said cheerfully, "in you go."

Tom was a little perplexed.

"Where are we going?"

"Down to X-ray. Way in the basement in the other building. I call it the dungeon

SAD BUT TRUE

48

Percentage of patients in the hospital whose understanding about what tests they were supposed to get was different from the orders their doctors had given

Study of 233 patients published in 2010 by the Mayo Clinic[137]

sometimes, it's so gloomy looking. They try to cheer it up by painting the walls bright colors, but it's still a dungeon to me."

"Okay, but why are we going there?"

"They want you to have a test."

"What kind of test?"

"Just says here to take you to X-ray. They know all about it. They'll take good care of you. You don't have to worry about a thing."

Reluctantly, Tom folded his newspaper and got into the wheelchair. The orderly greeted other employees cheerfully as he navigated a series of long corridors and two different elevators.

Tom was getting more and more concerned as the journey continued. His doctor hadn't talked about any more tests.

Finally, they arrived and the orderly said, "Now, don't you worry. When they're finished, they'll call up and you'll get me or somebody else to come take you back to your room."

Tom wasn't worried about getting back to his room. He was worried about the test. The technician started preparing to inject fluid into Tom's IV.

"Hold on there!" Tom said, alarmed. "What are you doing?"

"This is a contrast dye. It will help the doctor see what's going on inside you."

"I don't want this. I don't know what this test is or what it is for. My doctor didn't say anything about getting another test. I think this is a mistake."

"Oh, they don't always tell you what they're doing. It's a standard test."

"Do not put that dye into my arm. Stop right there. I want to know what this test is called, what it is for, and who authorized it. Don't come near me with that needle until you can tell me these things."

The technician sighed, put down the needle, and went to make a call.

He came back a few minutes later and said, "Oops! This test isn't for you after all. You're not supposed to have this test. I'll call Transport and have them come pick you up. You can wait right here until they come."

Tom's experience is not unusual.

How To Avoid Getting Tests by Mistake

1. **Agree to a plan for tests**.
   a. Ask your doctors to tell you the **names** of all tests they order for you.
   b. Ask the **purpose** of each one. (*You have a right to know what will be done to your body and why it is being done.*)
   c. If you have concerns about a test, ask if there are **other options**.
   d. Ask when tests you've agreed to are **scheduled**.

2. **Verify orders for tests you aren't expecting.**
   a. Ask to **see the order** that has your name on it.
   b. **Read it** carefully. (*Sometimes hospital employees accidentally mix up patients, especially if they have similar names.*)
   c. If the order is signed by a **doctor whose name you don't recognize**, that's a red flag.

3. **Refuse unexpected tests unless you can confirm that your doctor ordered them**.

SAD BUT TRUE

41-75

Percentage of patients who could not understand informed consent forms

Study reported in the Columbia University School of Nursing's "Health Literacy Overview"[138]

Recovering from surgery

Once care has been delivered, does the patient's need to know end? No, as Jack, age 54, discovered.

Jack lives in a suburb of Chicago and does fundraising for a non-profit. Some years ago, he was diagnosed with colon cancer and needed surgery to remove a section of his intestine.

Before the operation, he researched the surgery. He got personalized information when he met with the surgeon. The doctor did a great job explaining the tumor's location, its characteristics, and his plan for the operation. Everything proceeded as expected until the third day after surgery, when suddenly everything changed.

Jack recalled, "I was getting these tremendous pains in my abdomen. Remember the movie Alien *where the little monster jumps out of the guy's stomach? Well, that's what I felt like. I thought all these staples were going to go bing, bing, bing to the other side of the room, and this little monster was coming out of my stomach."*

Jack pressed the call button. The nurse arrived promptly and asked, "What's going on?" When Jack described the pain, the nurse explained exactly what was going on in Jack's colon.

"Three days after they reconnect your colon it decides to say, 'Well, you know, I think maybe I'll start trying to work.' They took out a 16" section of your colon. Now the two other pieces have been put back together. The one on the top is coming down saying, 'Okay, now I'm waiting for this next section to do what it's supposed to do,' but the next section isn't there. The lower section isn't quite ready to receive things because it's waiting for the missing piece, so there's this little tussle at the point of reconnection."

After he finished, he said, "No one's ever told you this?"

Jack felt a little silly for never having asked about recovery. He and the surgeon had both focused on what would happen during the operation.

He said, "That taught me a lesson. If I ever have to have something like this again, I'm going to ask, 'Now, what should I be expecting during my recovery?'"

How To Avoid Surprises After Surgery

1. **Ask what short-term downsides to expect.**
   a. What will happen during the surgery itself that might cause me **temporary problems** right afterwards? (*For example, will my throat be sore because I had a breathing tube? Will I have pain from gas pumped into my abdomen to separate organs?*)
   b. How much **pain** am I likely to have as a result of the surgery, and for how long?
   c. What **restrictions or limitations** will I have, and for how long?

2. **Ask when basic functions are likely to be possible:**
   a. **Eating** a normal diet.
   b. **Drinking** beverages you prefer.
   c. **Getting out of bed.**
   d. **Using the toilet** normally.

3. **Ask when more complex actions will be possible:**
   a. **Bathing normally.**
   b. **Having sex.**
   c. **Thinking clearly.**

4. **Ask what steps to take to aid in rapid recovery.**

5. **Clarify longer-term expectations.**
   a. When will I be able to **go back to work**?
   b. How long will it take before I am **back to normal**?
   c. Is the **new normal** going to be **like the old normal**, or will I have permanent changes to get used to?

SAD BUT TRUE

14

Percentage of information that doctors give orally during office visits that patients remember

Study on patient recall quoted in the *Journal of the Royal Society of Medicine*[139]

Jack reflected, "Had I known that three days after surgery I will probably experience this, my anxiety level would have been a lot lower. I still would have been in pain, and I probably would have been worried. I almost passed out. But at least I would have realized, 'They told me this might happen, and it is happening, so I guess it's probably okay.'"

Surprisingly alert despite the pain, Jack had the presence of mind to ask what would happen next. The nurse explained in detail the progress he could expect, leading to an almost full recovery 6-8 weeks later. Jack has now been cancer-free for more than five years, and he has become very practiced at asking questions of his doctors.

Remembering what the doctor said

Charles, legs dangling uncomfortably off the examination table, tried to pull the paper gown around himself, again, as the doctor was talking.

"Sally will give you your prescriptions when you check out. That's after you go down the hall to Juanita and get your blood drawn. Now, do those exercises every day. Oh, and pick up the referral from Miriam. Don't forget, I want to see you in two weeks."

Charles was cold. Looking forward to putting his clothes back on and going home, he tried to remember what Nancy had asked him to get at the store. Bananas and milk? Or milk and eggs?

"Any questions?"

"Uh . . . no, Doc, thanks."

Charles arrived home with bananas, milk, bread, and eggs, hoping that he had gotten what Nancy had asked for. She turned and smiled fondly at him as he walked into the kitchen.

"What did the doctor say?"

Charles glanced at the groceries, tried to recall, and then shrugged.

"Nothing, really."

Charles is fictional, but his experience is common. Further, patients remember diagnoses far more often than they remember treatment plans.[140] Thus, they may not take the next steps that the doctor outlines, for the simple reason that they forget what they are.

Consider whether Charles was set up to succeed or set up to fail to remember what the doctor said.

First, he was uncomfortable. His legs were dangling, so he probably didn't feel stable. He was cold and had to use one or both hands to hold the paper gown closed. These physical distractions took his attention away from the doctor's words.

SAD BUT TRUE

40-80

Percentage of information doctors give that patients typically forget right away

❁

Study on patient recall quoted in the *Journal of the Royal Society of Medicine*[141]

Second, he may have felt embarrassed or exposed, a common reaction when someone in authority is fully clothed and the less powerful person in the room is naked or nearly so. This emotional distraction can make it hard to concentrate.

Third, while the doctor doubtless had a computer, a pen, and documents, Charles didn't. Even if he had brought a pad of paper and a pen, he couldn't get to them when he was on an elevated exam table, his belongings across the room on a chair. Charles couldn't take a single note—and he's the one who was expected to complete multiple action steps. This logistical barrier made it hard to keep track of all the instructions the doctor gave.

Have you ever met someone who says, "Give me a call and we'll do lunch," when you both know that he has an unlisted number that he hasn't given you? You know right away that he doesn't really expect you to call him. If you are in Charles' shoes, you can be forgiven for believing that the doctor doesn't really expect you to remember what he's said; the circumstances make it very difficult to do so, a fact that is surely obvious to everyone.

See the boxes on the next two pages for simple steps the doctor and patient can take to help the patient recall the doctor's instructions.

How Doctors Can Help Improve Patient Recall

1. **Give patients a clipboard, a pen, and a blank form**.
    For use during the visit, the form can list fill-in-the-blank
    sentences that answer common questions. For example,
    some of the lines might read:
    a. **"My diagnosis is** _____**."**
    b. **"I will have a test called** _____
        at _____ (location, time) **to find out**
        _____**."**
    c. **I will hear the results by** _____ (date)."

2. **Give patients handouts that use simple language,
    pictures, and graphics to explain key points.**

3. **Ask patients to explain their diagnoses and what
    they need to do.**
    This approach is one of the most successful.[142] (*For exam-
    ple, in Charles' case, the doctor might say, "Nancy is sure to
    ask you what I said. What will you tell her?"*)

4. **Give patients a printout with summary notes.**
    They can take home both their notes and the doctor's.
    The doctor's can list **symptoms**, **diagnoses, treatments,
    tests scheduled, test results reported**, and **next steps**.

5. **Remind the patient to take the documents home:**
    a. **Their completed form** from the clipboard.
    b. **Handouts that explain conditions or treatments.**
    c. The **printed summary of key facts from the visit.**

6. **Have a staff member call the patient to follow up.**
    Staff might call in one or two days to answer questions
    and clarify next steps.

How Patients Can Recall Instructions

1. **Prepare a list of questions to take with you.**
   Examples include:
   a. What is my **diagnosis**?
   b. What are the **names and doses of any drugs** that you are prescribing?
   c. **What is each drug for?**
   d. **What else do I need to do**?
   e. When should I **start to feel better**?
   f. When should I **come back**?

2. **Ask someone to come with you to take notes**.
   You might ask your spouse, another family member, or a friend.

3. **Take a pad of paper and a pen with you.**
   Doing so will allow you and/or your companion to take notes.

4. **Prepare your doctor to help you remember important information.**
   a. Ask to be given time to **get dressed** before the doctor gives instructions.
   b. Consider asking to **record the visit**, especially if you don't bring someone with you. (*Many smartphones can record; you may choose to download an app with additional recording features.*)
   c. Give the doctor a copy of your **list of questions**.

5. **Keep a copy of your questions and write down the doctor's answers on it.**
   It's fine if you and your companion both write down information. Doing so makes it less likely that key points will be missed.

SAD BUT TRUE

Half

Proportion of information that patients recall from office visits that they remember incorrectly

Study on patient recall quoted in the *Journal of the Royal Society of Medicine*[143]

Notice that many of the changes suggested are relatively easy, quick, and inexpensive to make. (Handing the patient a printout summarizing the visit does assume that the doctor is using electronic medical records; other action steps do not.)

Why isn't it common practice to take steps like these?

If the point of an office visit is simply for the doctor to create records and bill the insurance company—that is, if the purpose of the visit is achieved shortly after the patient walks out the door—then it doesn't matter if the patient remembers what was said.

But imagine instead that the purpose of the office visit is to create a step-by-step plan that everyone with a role to play can follow, to help resolve a medical problem that is interfering with the patient's ability to lead the life he wants. In that case, it's critical that patients retain clear and accurate memories of every single point in the plan. However, Charles and his doctor both acted as if the patient *doesn't* need to know what's going on.

9

"Medical records are for doctors"

From medical test results to doctors' notes, records about your health may be invisible to you, because medical professionals often are the only ones who see them. You could be harmed or even die needlessly if your medical records contain critical information that you haven't heard about, or contain mistakes that lead to treatment errors.

Delayed reporting of test results

Two or three months after starting treatment for multiple sclerosis (MS), Shannon felt more exhausted than ever. In a routine check-up in early April, the neurologist ran blood tests to rule out any unknown problems.

Later that month, Shannon dragged herself out of bed and put on a smiling face to lead a team of friends on a three-mile MS walkathon. They all walked at a casual stroll, worried about Shannon's energy level. Even so, Shannon and her walking partner fell further and further behind as Shannon struggled simply to keep putting one foot in front of the other.

Convinced that the overwhelming exhaustion would be part of her life from now on, Shannon shifted back and forth between despair and acceptance. In late May, she saw the neurologist for another six-week checkup. The next day, she got a call telling her to return to the doctor's office right away.

When she arrived, the doctor explained that her blood test results from six weeks earlier had shown a condition called pancytopenia: she had a dangerously low level of red blood cells, white blood cells, and platelets in her blood.

The situation was a medical emergency, but no one had told Shannon or ordered any treatment. The previous day, six weeks after the earlier tests, another round of blood tests revealed an even further dramatic drop in all three components of her blood.

The doctor was very upset and wanted to put Shannon in the hospital right away to give her blood transfusions and monitor her condition.

Why had no one said anything six weeks earlier? Shannon had two doctors, her primary care doctor and the neurologist specializing in MS. The neurologist had ordered the test, and the results were sent to both doctors. Each assumed that the other would follow up.

Instead, Shannon had endured grueling exhaustion, emotional torment, and very serious changes in her blood for much longer than necessary, simply because her doctors did not notify her promptly of the first test results.

Stress from delays

The federal government has ruled that patients must be given ready access to their medical test results starting in October 2014.[145] Historically, though, people usually could not get test results until the doctor agreed to release them. Why not? Doctors argued that patients wouldn't know how to interpret them and might become upset and confused.[146]

Making people wait for their test results implies that people are less distressed by waiting than they are by getting the test results promptly from the testing service or from a staff member in the doctor's office.

That is a questionable assumption for three reasons. First, people in situations like Shannon's prefer to find out quickly that they have a life-threatening problem. Second, most tests are done to rule out problems, and that's exactly what they do. Most people are relieved, not upset or confused, by the results. The issue of false positives can be addressed with clear communication.[147]

Third, research shows that uncertainty all by itself is harmful. Even people with cancer would be better off knowing as soon as possible.

A Harvard researcher concluded, "Human beings find uncertainty more painful than the things they're uncertain about. . . . An uncertain future leaves us stranded in an unhappy present with nothing to do but wait."[148]

A *New York Times* article described the experience of one woman waiting for cancer test results, which her doctor had promised to get to her in the two days before he left on an extended vacation: "Racing pulse, dry mouth, total self-preoccupation with what-ifs to the point that real life doesn't exist, willing the phone to ring."

When she hadn't heard from the doctor on the first day, she left messages begging him to call. The second day, she waited by the phone, "'jumping at every noise, not letting anyone use the phone, imagining every scenario.' Her doctor left for his vacation. He never called, not even when he returned."[150]

Stress can actually injure the human body on the cellular level and speed up aging.[151] In fact, Dr. Elizabeth Blackburn, who was awarded a Nobel prize for her work on the impact of stress on aging and disease, noted, "Relieving patient stress . . . is looking more and more important."[152]

Interacting with patients in ways deliberately designed to *decrease* their stress levels—rather than unthinkingly *increase* them—might be one of the best ways that doctors could contribute to their patients' health. Since not knowing medical test results causes high stress levels, and high stress levels damage health, one way to have test results enhance rather than harm people's health is to provide them as quickly as possible.

One doctor, interviewed by *WebMD* about this picture, said, "The big-

> **SAD BUT TRUE**
>
> # 55-71
>
> Percentage of doctors who say they always tell patients about their *abnormal* test results
>
>
>
> Study involving 148 doctors, published in the *Journal of General Internal Medicine*[149]

SAD BUT TRUE

0-26

Percentage of seriously abnormal test results that doctors did not report to patients

❀

Study in the *Archives of Internal Medicine* involving 1,889 seriously abnormal results handled by more than 105 physicians; on average, doctors failed to notify patients 7 percent of the time[154]

gest mistake we see when we see these things not dealt with is when the doctor knows the patient has an appointment in a month and plans to deal with it then, and then the patient doesn't show up."[153]

Notice two implications: first, it's fine to wait a month to tell people their test results; second, if doctors don't provide the results even after a month, it's the patient's fault.

The *WebMD* article continued, "And in many cases, doctors may choose not to call patients 'because we know that they know we know what's going on, and they trust us, so we don't call unless it's necessary,' he says. 'We have found when we call patients about lab results, they give us better patient satisfaction scores. But we don't want to call with information that could confuse them, give them more information than they need for some minor change. You can create anxiety. If the result is expected or not relevant, we don't call.'"[155]

Notice that the doctor, knowing which approach leads to higher patient satisfaction, has decided that doing the *opposite* is best for them.

If you never hear the test results, what happens to your stress levels?

Sleeping Beauty's test results

When might people be better off not getting test results promptly or not getting them at all? The most likely answer is: when they have no idea what they are being tested for and so aren't concerned about the results. But that scenario implies giving up bodily fluids or tissue samples or undergoing other tests without being given any reason.

If people are expected to be intelligent consumers of health care, they need to know the purpose of any proposed test and agree to it, and thus they will know what it might reveal. For example, if they are being tested for diabetes, then they know that the test might indicate that they have diabetes.

To conclude that it doesn't matter when—or if—you get your test results, doctors would have to believe that you are in a state of suspended animation, with no thoughts or feelings at all about the tests you've had, unless and until the doctor interacts with you—just as Sleeping Beauty is dead to the world until the prince kisses her.

Errors in medical records common

Test results are one type of medical record. Your doctor keeps many others. It's important to know what those records say, partly because they often contain mistakes.

SAD BUT TRUE

Equal

Stress levels in women told that they had breast cancer and stress levels in women still waiting for their breast cancer test results after five days

Harvard research comparing cortisol (stress hormone) levels in 16 women told they had cancer, 37 told they didn't, and 73 still waiting for their test results[156]

Janice and her doctor discussed whether it would be medically useful for her to have an indoor swimming pool. Later, she saw in her medical records a summary of that conversation: "The patient would like to have a laparoscopic cholecystectomy in her house."

A laparoscopic cholecystectomy is an operation to remove a gall bladder. Janice's doctor is keenly intelligent, and Janice is very glad to be his patient. But her gallbladder is in excellent condition, and they certainly never discussed having it removed in her house.

When she called, the doctor's assistant was completely unapologetic about the error. Janice and her doctor had discussed a "lap pool." The first three letters of that phrase are the same as the first three letters of "laparoscopic cholecystectomy." The doctor's office uses a computer program to transcribe his recorded notes. It includes a "type ahead" feature—when it knows the first few letters of a word or phrase, it guesses what the rest will be, based on terms commonly used in the doctor's practice. Evidently, more people talk to the doctor about having their gallbladders out than about getting swimming pools.

Doctors' reluctance to give access

An equally big problem is that people often find it challenging to find out what is in their medical records in the first place.

One study said, "Patients have little access to information and knowledge that can help them participate in, let alone guide, their own care." Patients at least need access to their doctors' records showing "their own diagnoses, medications, allergies, lab test results, visit summaries, and other findings over time."[158]

Some doctors oppose computerizing records, worried that patients might then be able to access them more easily. If records are going to be electronic, doctors suggested that they would put less information in them, so that patients wouldn't be able to see what they were thinking.[159]

Imagine a professional football team whose players don't know the game scores or their own statistics. They don't see game films, much less review them with coaches to analyze what worked and what didn't.

Imagine also that coaches say that they don't give players a lot of information because it would just upset or confuse them. The coaches also don't track whether the plays they call work or not, and a lot of their coaching consists of telling players, "You need to do a better job playing football."

How would you rate their chances of getting to the Super Bowl?

You probably wouldn't want to bet on that.

Now imagine a health care system in which patients have trouble getting their own medical records. They don't have a debriefing after treatment to discuss whether it improved their lives or not.

Imagine also that doctors say that they don't give patients a lot of information because it would just upset or confuse them. The doctors also don't track whether the treatments they prescribe improve people's lives. A lot of their advice consists of telling patients, "You need to do a better job taking care of yourself."

How would you rate the chances of getting great results from a health care system like that?

You probably wouldn't want to bet on that either. Yet that's the health care system most people in the United States experience today.

Wouldn't it be great if you could have access to all your medical records online, just as you can access all your Amazon.com orders? You might consider this idea a no-brainer. The health care profession doesn't.

> **SAD BUT TRUE**
>
> # 1 in 4
>
> People who found errors in their medical records when they had the opportunity to review them
>
>
>
> Study in the *Journal of the American Medical Informatics Association*; electronic records, increasingly common, can increase the number of errors[160]

In a year-long study by the Harvard Medical School, many doctors assumed that their workload would increase if patients had ready access to their records, because they thought they would have to spend a great deal of time explaining the contents and calming anxious or distressed patients.

As is typically the case when professionals predict dire problems when patients are allowed to engage more in their own care, "Their fears simply never materialized."[161]

Instead, doctors found that "there was more trust, better communication, more shared decision-making and increased patient satisfaction." Patients "felt more in control of their own care" and most reported that "reading their doctors' notes helped them to take their medications more regularly and better follow their doctors' treatment recommendations."[162]

What difference does it make to your health and your care if you don't see your medical records? If you don't know what tests you've had, what the results were, what conclusions doctors have drawn, and so forth, you may make mistakes in caring for yourself, and you also can't clearly explain your medical history to the next doctor you see.

Your doctors may order duplicate tests, misdiagnose you, prescribe

SAD BUT TRUE

94

Percentage of people who believe that they should be able to access their own medical records online (but see box on facing page)

❀

Harvard Medical School study of 105 doctors and 13,564 patients over the course of a year, reported in 2012 in the *Annals of Internal Medicine* [163]

treatments that harmed you before, and miss important problems. They may fail to connect the dots because they don't have the whole story.

When doctors send each other copies of your records, they may base their conclusions and actions on errors that go unchecked—because you may be the only person who would notice the mistakes. In Janice's case, doctors might assume that she needed her gall bladder removed and that only the suggestion that it be done at home was wrong.

Despite these issues, many doctors still don't want patients to see their own charts. One doctor said, "I think it would be—at best an inconvenience for me that I would no longer feel comfortable putting down: 'There's a distant possibility of a brain tumor. If the headaches are still going on two weeks from now, let's get a CT scan.'" [164] Building on that example, imagine that your symptoms worsen, and you end up in the emergency room at two a.m. on a Sunday.

Your not knowing what your doctor is thinking doesn't help you get better care. It endangers your life. Misdiagnosis rates in the ER run as high as 40 percent. [165] The less information you can contribute, the greater the chance that harried ER staff will miss something important. The doctor isn't with you 24 hours a day, 7 days a week, to provide information about your medical history. The only person there all the time is you.

Despite the benefits of having people review their medical records, some professionals try to steer you towards Personal Health Records (PHRs) instead. These are records you keep, in order to track "daily symptoms, over-the-counter medicines taken, personal exercise programs, special diets, or data from home monitoring devices." [166]

That information can be very useful. However, the traditional hard-core medical data, such as the results of tests and physical exams, would remain in the Electronic Medical Record (EMR), the province of doctors. In some cases, individuals may be given limited access to part of their EMR, but be blocked from seeing other parts, such as the doctor's notes.

Getting copies of medical records

Until all your health records are available electronically to you and to any doctor or hospital that might treat you, creating your own PHR is one of the most useful steps you can take to manage your health.

As used here, the term PHR is meant to be comprehensive, including not only information that you create, such as notes about symptoms you have, but also information from people or organizations that have tested or treated you (for example, doctors, labs, and hospitals).

SAD BUT TRUE

Up to 80

Percentage of doctors who said they were "frightened" by the idea of allowing patients access to their own medical records online

❀

Harvard Medical School study of 105 doctors and 13,564 patients over the course of a year, reported in 2012 in the *Annals of Internal Medicine*[167]

The first step is to decide what records you need. Since collecting all of them can seem like a daunting task, start with this more hopeful thought: any records you get will put you in a better position than you are now.

For non-life-threatening issues, you might seek just the most recent few years of records. Care providers can charge by the page, so you might skip older records unless you think that they might change your care today. If you don't remember the names of doctors or testing sites you've been to, your insurer's Explanation of Benefits forms may help.

One category of records to collect relates to health issues that interfere with your ability to lead the life you want. For example, if you would dearly love to keep up with your grandchildren, but you have asthma that seriously slows you down, you might seek records related to your breathing problems. Do allergies trigger asthma attacks, which in turn set the stage for bronchitis? Is your breathing getting better or worse over time? Which treatments have helped? Which have not? This information can help you better manage your condition.

A second category of records to get concerns major medical events such as heart attacks or surgery; doctors will often ask you about these.

Don't assume that you'll always be able to get such records in the future if you need them. Doctors may dispose of your records when a certain amount of time has passed since they last saw you; the term varies by state, but is often six or seven years.

A third category of records to get relates to chronic conditions that require ongoing management, such as diabetes or heart disease, even if these are currently well controlled.

You might ask for all records including test results, doctors' notes, and write-ups about x-rays or other diagnostic tests, but excluding the images themselves. Unless you need to take the images to another doctor, getting these special types of records may simply add time and cost without changing the care you get.

If you are seeking one piece of information such as a test result related to a recent office visit, call and ask for it. If you want more (or older) records, you will probably need to put your request in writing. You have a legal right to see your medical records (with some exceptions related to mental illness and substance abuse.)

The steps to get your records vary a little by state. Search online for [medical record rights in (name of state where you got care)]. State governments usually post information that explains how to proceed. A box at the end of the chapter provides typical requirements. Steps are similar whether you are asking for records from doctors, from hospitals, or from other sites.

Generally, doctors and others must provide these records within 30 days, but some states mandate a faster turnaround. State websites will usually tell you how to complain if you haven't been able to get your records in a timely manner after providing all the necessary information.

A doctor's office might ask why you want the records, so that they know what to give you. For instance, if you are getting a second opinion from another surgeon, you will probably need to take copies of your actual x-rays.

Sometimes, though, the question is a throwback to days when people typically asked for records only if they were going to sue or switch doctors. It is perfectly acceptable to say simply, "I am getting copies of all my medical records for my personal files."

Reviewing your medical records

What should you do with your records once you have them?

First, know that you may want to give a copy of your records to other doctors in the future. That copy should *not* have any notes you make on it. For this reason, either make a copy of the copy to write your comments and questions on, or use sticky notes that you can remove.

Second, as you begin to read the records, start by assuming that your doctors are simply doing their jobs and realize that it may be easy to misinterpret their notes. For example, "SOB" is not an insult. It stands for Short of Breath. Either look up abbreviations on a reputable website, or ask someone knowledgeable to translate.

Third, if you are attempting to unravel a medical mystery, note anything you find in the records that you didn't already know or that doesn't seem to match the facts you do know.

Fourth, if your medical situation is complicated, create a chronological summary that uses just a few lines per interaction to capture key data:

- the date
- the name of the doctor or other provider
- the reason for the contact
- tests and their results
- diagnoses
- treatments
- other conclusions/comments/next steps

At first glance, the diagnoses you have been given may not be obvious. If you see DX or DX1, DX2, and so forth, followed by several numbers, the doctor has used codes to capture your diagnoses.

To find out what the numbers mean, go to http://www.icd9data. com/2014/Volume1/default.htm and type into the search box the numbers you found in your records, for example, 493 or 493.82. Doctors sometimes write down two or more diagnostic codes; look them all up. (Ignore the ads on the website, which sometimes highlight scary medical problems.)

Even complex medical situations can often be summarized as described above in just a few pages, useful to give to any new doctor you see.

Fifth, once you have combed through your records for surprises and have prepared a summary of your medical history, you might put together a list of questions for your doctor and/or a list of other actions to take. For example, you might realize that you never heard back about a recent test. You might realize that you are still taking a drug for a condition you no longer have. You may see notes about plans for follow-ups that sound unfamiliar.

Correcting errors in your medical records

One medical records expert noted that errors in medical records "happen all the time."[169] It helps to understand what is considered an error and what isn't. Examples of entries in your medical records that would *not* be considered mistakes follow:

- Diagnoses you object to (for example, depression or obesity).
- The doctor's conclusions that offend you (such as the need to lose weight or do a better job managing stress).
- The doctor's data (for example, your weight according to his scale).

Examples of entries that *would* be considered mistakes follow:

- "Left leg amputation," when both legs are intact.
- "Treated for depression for ten years," when the period was two years.
- "Complained of abdominal pain," when pain wasn't discussed.
- "Reports improvement," when the patient reported further decline.
- "Will start Drug X," when the patient did not agree to do so.
- Conclusions that are incorrect, such as that a patient has allergies because she reported taking a certain allergy medicine, when in fact the drug was prescribed to treat an inner ear balance problem.
- Data that clearly describe a different patient.
- Typos in diagnostic code numbers, such as recording 340 (multiple sclerosis) when they meant 640 (bleeding during pregnancy).

You might be surprised to learn that erroneous information can't actually be removed from your records. For legal reasons, once a record is created, it is as if it were cast in stone. Instead, records can be "amended," which means adding a statement describing the error and giving the correct information.

To amend your record, you will need to put your request in writing. Include the exact language that you want your doctor to put into the medical record. It needs to be reasonable and appropriate to the situation. For example, it won't help to write, "You didn't listen to me at all the last time I was in. You need to change my medical record and take back those things you said I told you, because I didn't say any of that."

It is more useful to write, "I ask that you amend your notes from my visit to you on June 26, 2014. Your notes say that I said that I had insomnia, stomachaches, and diarrhea every day for the preceding two months. Please add the following statement to my records: "The patient notes that she did not have insomnia, a stomachache, and diarrhea every day for the preceding two months. She notes that she had these symptoms for a total of two days in the preceding two months, and that they resolved on their own without any treatment.'"

Interestingly, it is not enough to ask that your records be amended simply because they are wrong. You typically must explain why you believe the error needs to be addressed. In this example, you might say, "I would like you to amend my record because I am concerned that other doctors who see those records may conclude that I have a serious chronic gastrointestinal problem when I don't."

Generally, the only doctor who can correct an error in your records is the one who created it. If Doctor A created medical records with an error in them and then sent copies of your file to Doctors B, C, and D, there is no point in asking Doctor B, C, or D to correct the record.

Search on [amend medical records in (name of state)] for details about the process, including how long the doctor has to amend your records and what to do if the doctor fails to do so.

Tracking care events in real time

It will be easier in the future to know that you have a complete picture of your medical history if you begin to keep track as care takes place.

Examples of activities to include are a visit to a doctor, a dentist, or an eye care provider (whether a doctor or not); a flu shot at a local drugstore; a visit to other providers such as a chiropractor or acupuncturist; a medical test; a hospital stay; phone calls with any of the above people or organizations; and any other interaction with the health care system.

The information to capture is very similar to the information you extracted from your medical records to create a historical summary:

- Contact information for the doctor, hospital, and so forth.
- Reason for the visit/call.
- Tests done.
- Diagnoses you are given.
- Medicines prescribed, with the spelling of the name, the strength, dosing instructions, and the expected duration, such as 500 mg 4 times a day for 10 days.
- Next steps (what they are going to do, when you will hear back about test results, when you are supposed to go back, who else you are supposed to see, and so forth).

Add any other data not listed here that you feel is relevant to your care. It is helpful to take the folder/printout or relevant sections of your PHR when you see a doctor, enter the hospital, or have any other significant encounter with the health care system.

With your medical record in hand, you can be a more active player in your own care and health management, and you may save yourself from grave harm.

How To Get Your Medical Records

Ask if the doctor has a form you can fill out to request your records. If so, use it. Otherwise, ask what information they need to have in a letter from you. Generally, items will include:

1. **Identifying information:**
   a. The current **date**.
   b. Your **name**, **mailing address**, and **phone**.
   c. The **doctor's name** and **mailing address**.
   d. Your **Social Security number** or a medical record number, if they have assigned one to you.
   e. Your **date of birth**.

2. **Details of your inquiry:**
   a. A **request to release your medical records** to you, and the format you prefer (*such as paper, or electronic if available and paper if not, and so forth*).
   b. The **medical condition** for which you were seen, if you want just a subset of your records.
   c. The range of **dates** for which you want records (*such as May-July 2014*).
   d. The **records you are requesting** (*all records, specific test results, actual x-ray images, other diagnostic imaging, and so forth*).

3. **Agreement to pay.**
   The office should tell you the cost per page, but you won't know the total until after they have printed the records. They will also typically add a postage charge. Note **how you will pay** (*via check or credit card, for example*).

4. **Your signature.**

What To Do With Your Medical Records

1. **Prepare to review.**
    a. **Make a second copy** to write on, or get sticky notes on which to record any questions or comments.
    b. Start by assuming that everything in **your record is intended to help** get you better care.

2. **Read through the records and note key points**:
    a. Anything that **surprises** or alarms you.
    b. Any **errors.**
    c. Other **items to discuss** with your doctor (*such as care plans you didn't know about*).

3. **Summarize each contact with the health care system, in order by date.**
    Include (*on one or a few lines*):
    a. The **date** of the event.
    b. The **name** of the doctor, lab, hospital, or other.
    c. The **reason** for the contact (*for example, to report symptom xyz*).
    d. Names of **tests and their results**.
    e. **Diagnoses** you were given.
    f. **Drugs prescribed**, including the doses and how often each was to be taken.
    g. Other **treatments** you were given.
    h. Other important **conclusions** or comments.
    i. **Next steps**, including what they were, who was to take them, and by when.

4. **Organize the records for future reference.**

5. **Make any appointments needed.**

How To Correct Your Medical Records

Steps to amend your records are similar to steps to get your records. If the doctor has a form you can fill out, use that. Otherwise, ask what information they need to have in a letter from you. Generally, items will include:

1. **Identifying information:**
    a. The current **date**.
    b. Your **name**, **mailing address**, and **phone**.
    c. The **doctor's name** and **mailing address**.
    d. Your **Social Security number** or a medical record number, if they have assigned one to you.
    e. Your **date of birth**.

2. **Details of your request:**
    a. The fact that **you are asking that they amend** your medical records.
    b. The **date of the error**, **type of record** that contains the error (*for example, doctor's notes or lab test*), and a **clear description** of the mistake.
    c. The **statement you have crafted** that you want them to add to the record (*see text*).
    d. **Why the record needs to be corrected.**

3. **Your signature.**

Once your doctor has amended your records:

4. **Request a copy of the amended record.**

5. **Request that corrected copies be sent out.**
    a. Put your **request in writing**.
    b. Ask that the amended record be sent to **specific doctors you name** who you believe received the erroneous information.

10

"Doctor knows best"

Dr. Peter Pronovost, a leader in improving patient care, commented, "In every hospital in America, patients die because of hierarchy." He explained that doctors say to nurses, in effect, "I'm right. I'm more senior than you. Don't tell me what to do."[170]

What Dr. Pronovost didn't mention is that patients occupy an even lower rung on the ladder than nurses do. They often have no seat at the table, no voice in their own care. In some cases, doctors may use their authority to order tests and treatments to make money, rather than to help the patient.

A paradoxical reaction

Terry had been thrown many times while horseback riding—once breaking her thighbone in four places. She'd been riding rogue horses most of her life. But she finds dealing with the health care system much scarier than riding wild horses.

When she broke her wrist one weekend five years ago in another horse-riding accident, she didn't want to waste money on the emergency room. Instead, she wrapped her wrist and waited until Monday to see a doctor.

He told her that she'd never work again or ride another wild horse—if he didn't operate on her wrist right away. Terry was a truck driver and a construction worker, and she needed the use of both of her hands and arms. She was scared by his dramatic pronouncement.

SAD BUT TRUE

10

Percentage of patients who reported that their doctors mentioned any alternative to the treatment that they (doctors) recommended

❁

Study published in 2012 in the *Journal of General Internal Medicine* involving 472 patients who got stents implanted (when researchers considered several other treatment options to be equally valid)[171]

She reluctantly agreed to the surgery—but explained that she has what is called a "paradoxical reaction" to any drug that affects her mental state. When she had been given anesthesia on two prior occasions, she had awakened shouting and swinging, ripping out IV lines and throwing things.

She was very emphatic: no anesthesia, no drugs that would impact her mental state; she wanted to remain conscious and alert during the procedure. She asked to have only a nerve block, injections into her arm to prevent pain signals from reaching her brain.

After she finished, the doctor stopped talking about anesthesia.

Terry commented, "I thought that was settled, but it turns out that I might as well have been talking to my bedroom wall."

Among the dozen or so people who trooped in and out of her room the night before the surgery was a nurse anesthetist. But he didn't introduce himself or explain his role. Terry didn't realize that his breezy, "How's it going? Any questions?" marked her last chance to talk about the plan.

The next morning, the nurse anesthetist prepared to administer anesthesia. Terry, startled, said again that she did not want anesthesia because of her paradoxical reaction to it. The nurse anesthetist then called for a shot of Vitamin V.

"Vitamin V?" Terry asked, confused. "What are you talking about?"

"Oh, it's just to help relax your muscles, nothing to worry about."

Terry remembers thinking, Boy, I hope this isn't like calling a giant guy "Tiny," and this is some vitamin that will knock me on my keister. *Minutes later, she watched in horror as the nurse anesthetist continued to prepare the anesthesia.*

He said, "I think I know what's best for you; you're just a truck driver."

Terry found herself unable to argue. Later, she discovered that the reference to Vitamin V was code for Versed, a drug sometimes given before surgery to reduce anxiety and foster amnesia. For Terry, it didn't have that effect.

"I was angry when they knocked me out. I was livid. [But] I couldn't move. I was just like an amoeba, and I obeyed every command. What I wanted to do was jump off the table and storm out. But this drug makes you very uncoordinated. I just couldn't do anything. I was helpless."

After the surgery, Terry recalled, *"I woke up screaming and fighting in the recovery room. I was on my feet, in and out of consciousness, throwing things and hitting people."*

They tried to give her pain medicine, but she wasn't aware of pain. She was enraged. She shouted, *"You had no right to give me general anesthesia against my will!"*

"We gave you a little something to give you amnesia. You can't possibly remember what went on."

But she did.

She reported, *"I felt completely demoralized, humiliated, angry. I wanted to kill the certified nurse anesthetist. Seriously, if he had been there I would have lunged for his throat. And I'm just not like that, but I was absolutely beside myself. I was going in and out of consciousness. They wanted me out of there. They said, 'Shh. What about the other patients?' My husband said when I had the blackouts I was swearing like a sailor. He was afraid."*

The drug Terry was given *"can produce a wide variety of abnormal mental responses and very hazardous behavioral abnormalities: rebound anxiety, insomnia, psychosis, paranoia, violence, antisocial acts, depression, and suicide."*[173]

Such drugs *"can occasionally cause apparently paradoxical stimulation with increased aggression [and] anger."*[174] This reaction is more common in *"action-oriented individuals,"*[175] which Terry clearly is.

"My theory is that the drug shut down part of my brain that I tried desperately to reinstate, and there's like a rebound when the drug clears your system. I was so anxious [after the surgery]. I was crazy, and I felt like I was crazy, and there was nothing I could do. It felt like somebody had short-circuited my head."

Over the next few days, Terry remained severely upset. *"I couldn't sleep. I was*

SAD BUT TRUE

19

Percentage of patients who said that their doctors mentioned any possible downsides (risks) of the treatment they recommended

❈

Study published in 2012 in the *Journal of General Internal Medicine* involving 472 patients who got stents implanted[172]

SAD BUT TRUE

40

Percentage of patients who agreed that the informed consent form they signed reflected their understanding of the treatment's risks and benefits

Analysis referenced on the website of the American Academy of Orthopaedic Surgeons in 2013[176]

crying all the time. . . . I just went berserk. I couldn't do anything but cry and make complaints. . . . I was just crazy." Terry wryly noted that before surgery, her chart reported that she was "a very pleasant woman in no distress."

Complications

Terry also suffered a number of complications from the surgery itself. For example, the screws that the surgeon had put in stuck up and pressed against tendons and nerves, causing extreme pain. When she called to complain, the surgeon "fired" her as a patient.

Terry was nevertheless too scared to go to another doctor for a year and a half. Then, the doctor she saw "said the screws should be taken out immediately if not sooner, that it was completely unacceptable the way it was."

But red flags went up when the doctor said that he was sure that the surgery had been done correctly and that the only reason the screws were sticking out now was that her bone must have shrunk. Terry had x-rays showing that the screws had been sticking out from the beginning. She didn't want to entrust her body to someone who deliberately misled her.

"The second doctor, who lied to me, was very fatherly. He was a wonderful person, very soothing. I really liked him. But I don't want to be treated like a child. How I deal with things, I want to deal with it head on. Obviously the first surgery was poorly done. I don't want you to say, 'It's terrible right now, but it probably was perfect when he did it. It's just one of those things.' That doesn't make me feel better."

She said with regret, "Even though I really liked his bedside manner, I wish he hadn't said that. How can you trust him? You don't know these people. You trust them because they have vastly superior education in the medical field than you do, but I'm just not feeling the love. We need to meet in the middle like any negotiation. It's not just I go in there, 'Please help me. I'm so helpless. Do whatever you want.' No, we're going to negotiate this like adults. And it is my body. I live with it. You don't. He lied to me, so I went to another doctor and just said, 'Take them out.' I said, 'No Versed! No anesthesia!' They did it the way I told them to. They wanted to argue with me over it, and I was very firm."

For years after being given drugs against her will, Terry experienced uncontrollable rage and post-traumatic stress disorder (PTSD). She said sadly, "My daughter tells me that her mother left home that day and it took years for me to come back. My daughter was seven years old."

Terry was told that she was solely responsible for the problems she experienced. The anesthesiologist supervising the nurse anesthetist told her, "You must have been insane to start with."

Recently, Terry said, "PTSD is subsiding over time. I can sleep at night now. I still tend to be more irritable, quicker to anger. [But] it is getting better."

SAD BUT TRUE

26

Percentage of "informed consent" forms that contained four required elements: description of the treatment, its risks, its benefits, and alternatives

Research study mentioned in 2013 on the website of the Agency for Healthcare Research and Quality, U.S. Department of Health & Human Services[177]

Terry still suffers: "I get flashbacks. I get nervous and sweaty. I can't drive past the hospital." She faces skepticism from people who are certain that the drugs she was given cannot cause side effects. "They can't believe it. I would never have believed it [myself]. My story would be unbelievable to me if I hadn't lived through it." Since then, she has found an online community of people with similar experiences.

Terry agreed to the original surgery only because the doctor said that she wouldn't have full use of her hand and arm without it. But five years later, she still has regained only about 30 percent of the use of that arm. She reports, "I can work, but I can't climb ladders anymore. I can't hold wrenches. I've pretty much given up riding aggressive horses, because I just can't hold on."

Based on a review of her pre-surgical x-rays, another surgeon concluded that her wrist probably would have healed without any nerve damage or permanent disability if it had simply been put in a cast for six weeks, with no surgery at all. Terry is infuriated that scare tactics resulted in her getting a worse result than she probably would have gotten otherwise.

"I was just kept in the dark. . . . I can only assume that they felt if they gave me the true information that I would make the 'wrong' decision about what to do. I felt that I was conned. And then they chemically coerced me."

Avoiding health care to avoid its harm

The extreme distress has altered forever how Terry thinks about health care. The fact that a drug works well for the vast majority of people doesn't change the fact that it creates devastating problems for her. She worries that doctors will dismiss her medical history again in the future. She knows people whose doctors gave them the drug without their knowledge after they'd said that they had a bad re-action to it, to test that assertion.

She finds this possibility frightening, and it has changed how she lives her life.

"I used to love riding hunter/jumper horses. Not a chance now: I might injure myself and have to go to a doctor."

"Now I have a paranoia about being in a motor vehicle accident. I will not have a mammogram. I won't have any more pap smears. I will not be having a colo-noscopy, any of these diagnostics. Because my fear is they're going to tell me, 'There's a problem,' and they're going to send me to a hospital. And I don't think I can survive another thing like that. I totally lost my mind. I just can't face it."

Terry hopes that other people will learn from her experience.

One way to increase the odds that an unusual medical history will be believed is to provide your written medical records concerning the problem from the other doctors who treated you previously. Getting these documents added to Terry's file in the surgeon's office might have led him to take the issue seriously.

Terry pointed out that another defense is informed consent. If she had under-stood what the surgery entailed and its risks, she never would have agreed to have it.

"Read every single line there is on the intake paperwork and on the informed consent. Cross out things. They could refuse to treat you. That's the threat I lived with. They said, 'We just won't treat you if you don't allow us to do everything we have written on this sheet.' But that's not the law. You don't have to allow them to do any of this. You go through there and read it carefully, and don't let them rush you. If you have questions, talk to your surgeon."

She noted, "You need what they have to offer. But you have to figure out how to get what you want, as opposed to what they want to give you. You have to be brave enough and well enough to walk out. And that's huge. If you're sick and you're scared and your doctor is telling you, 'This is life-threatening,' you want to go along with whatever is going to save your life. You don't want him to say, 'Well, if you won't let me give you Versed, I won't treat you.' You don't want that. It's like a minefield. You have to be firm enough to where they don't do what you don't want. But you can't be firm and antagonize them, and some of them are easy to antagonize."

My way or the highway

Imagine a spouse who says, "I'll tell you what to do. If you disagree with me about anything, you can leave; we'll get a divorce." Does that sound like a relationship that would encourage you to ask questions and explore the pros and cons of different options?

Consider a doctor's comments: "The physician-patient compact basically states that a doctor will care for a patient in exchange for compensation and that the patient will heed the doctor's advice. Patients who disagree with their physicians . . . are free to go elsewhere."[179] Does *that* sound like a relationship that would encourage you to ask questions and explore the pros and cons of different options?

SAD BUT TRUE

16

Percentage of patients who reported that their doctors asked for their preferences when several good treatments were available

Study published in 2012 in the *Journal of General Internal Medicine* involving 472 patients who got stents implanted[178]

Prevention tells the story of a woman named Carla who was so gravely ill as a result of the thirteen prescription drugs she was taking that she felt she'd be better off dead. Her pharmacist prepared a carefully researched report showing that known side effects and drug interactions probably accounted for most of her symptoms.

When she gave the report to her doctor, he threw it across the room at her, saying, "I can't believe you'd insult me like this!" He then fired her as a patient. Notice his focus: she should not have questioned his authority.

Carla visited nine more doctors before finding one who would listen. The tenth doctor eliminated ten of the thirteen drugs; within weeks she felt "fifteen years younger" and continued to do well after that.[180]

No voice in treatment choices

An article in 2012 in the *New England Journal of Medicine* reported, "Patients and their families are often excluded from important discussions and left feeling in the dark about how their problems are being managed."[181]

The article suggested an idea still considered relatively daring in medical circles: doctors bring medical training and experience to the table, and patients bring their values and priorities. Then they use "shared decision-making" to jointly choose the treatment that suits the patient best.

However, doctors talking about this idea may subtly discredit patients and emphasize their own role.

Consider the only three concrete examples of shared decision-making described in one medical journal article on this topic: First, "the right of a competent adult to refuse a lifesaving blood transfusion." Second, "the right of a patient to refuse mechanical ventilation for a treatable and reversible cause of respiratory failure." Third, "patients' rights to demand care that physicians regard as medically inappropriate [such as] situations in which the likelihood of successful resuscitation would be less than 1 percent."

That is, all the concrete examples are about patients making choices that the doctor clearly viewed as irrational. He noted that health care has a history of benevolent paternalism. By implying that patients make only bad choices when given a say, he appeared to be justifying that stance.[182]

Involving patients in decisions about their care has been discussed—although not adopted—for many years; it is symbolized by the catch phrase, "Nothing about me without me," which started surfacing in 1998.[183]

In 1999, researchers concluded that patients have real choices only if they are asked which treatment they prefer after they understand five points:

- their right to have a say
- the nature of the medical issue involved
- their treatment options
- the pros and cons of each option
- the likelihood of success of each option[184]

Fifteen years later, studies continue to show that patients typically aren't given true choices.

Failing to make patients central

Shared decision-making is a basic building block of "patient-centered" care. "Patient-centered" care, one journal article explained, "seeks to focus medical attention on the individual patient's needs and concerns, rather than the doctor's."[185] But the physician who wrote that article inadvertently revealed his reluctance to give up a central role.

He compared doctor-centered health care to the ancient belief that the earth was the center of the universe and that the sun and the other planets revolved around it. In this analogy, the sun/patient orbits the earth/king/doctor. He then suggested the opposite, in which the earth/doctor orbits the sun/patient. Next he explained why, in his opinion, neither of these frameworks hits the mark.

"The flaw in the metaphor is that the patient and the doctor must coexist in a . . . relation of mutual and highly interwoven prerogatives. Neither is the king, and neither is the sun. Health relies on collaboration between the patient and the doctor. . . . Patient and physician must therefore meet as equals, bringing different knowledge, needs, concerns, and gravitational pull but neither claiming a position of centrality."

He went on, "A better metaphor might be a pair of binary stars orbiting a common center of gravity."[186]

Really?

What is the "common center of gravity" exerting a pull on both the doctor and the patient? The author did not say. He did not propose a larger cause such as public health, so set that possibility aside. What does occupy "a position of centrality" in medicine, if it is not meeting the patient's needs?

Consider an analogy. When building a home, most people hire a general contractor, who knows significantly more about building than homeowners do. Homeowners ignore the expert's advice at their peril. But that doesn't make the two parties equal players orbiting a third, unnamed player that they both serve. Both parties need to focus on identifying feasible solutions that will best meet the homeowners' needs. That's the point of the project.

People don't revere experts who claim that their own priorities are as important as those of the people they serve. People revere experts who do an outstanding job helping them to get their needs met.

Health care works best if doctors provide care that *enables people to lead the lives they want*. And that means involving patients—to the degree that they want to be involved—in creating care plans.

Discrimination: being treated as inferior

The day after Martin Luther King Jr. was shot in April 1968, Jane Elliott, a third-grade teacher in all-white Riceville, Iowa, decided to give her students a direct experience of discrimination.

She divided the class by eye color. The first day, blue-eyed children reigned supreme. She told the class that blue-eyed people were better, cleaner, and smarter. She gave them extra recess and first place in the lunch line. Brown-eyed children were not allowed to play with them.

Every time a blue-eyed child did something well, she used it as proof that all blue-eyed people are smarter and better than brown-eyed people. Every time a brown-eyed child did something less than perfectly, she used it as proof that all brown-eyed people are inferior.

The second day, she reversed the roles. The children got the message. Interestingly, their academic performance plummeted when they were treated as incompetent and inferior, and it soared when they were treated as intelligent and capable.[187]

Think about the impact on individuals who are routinely treated by the health care system as if they are incompetent and inferior even concerning topics on which they are the experts—their own symptoms and responses to treatment. Being discounted surely makes it harder for them to successfully manage their health and health care.

Being a good patient

Benjamin, age 28, woke up one Monday morning to find that he had severely swollen ankles and calves. In fact, the swelling extended almost to his knees. He told his wife, Theresa, "I am in heart failure." She thought he was too young for that, but did know that he had been fatigued since getting a cold several weeks earlier.

Benjamin's doctor took his blood pressure, but didn't look at his legs or examine him further. Benjamin had recently stopped smoking; his doctor said that swelling was his body's reaction to nicotine withdrawal and that his blood pressure was 180/100 only because he was anxious about seeing the doctor.

Hearing this report, Theresa, age 23, was furious and asked why Benjamin hadn't protested.

Benjamin said sincerely, "I was being a good patient. Good patients just do what they're told."

On Tuesday, Benjamin began vomiting clear water-like fluid, but the doctor's office said that they couldn't see him again until Wednesday. In that visit, they found that Benjamin had gained 20 pounds since Monday and that his blood pressure had continued to climb.

Theresa presented the doctor with a timeline laying out Benjamin's symptoms. The doctor ordered some tests and sent the couple home, still without thoroughly examining Benjamin.

The doctor's office called later that day. Benjamin's heart was enlarged to three times its normal size, and his blood tests also were abnormal. The doctor made an appointment for him to see a heart specialist on Friday. By then, Benjamin's blood pressure was even higher and he had gained much more weight.

The cardiologist took one look at his x-rays and blood tests and sent him to the Intensive Care Unit (ICU). He was suffering from heart, kidney, and liver failure and nearly died. He had only 5 percent of normal heart function, and it looked as if he might need a heart transplant.

He was retaining fluid because his kidneys were shutting down, and vomiting was his body's way of trying to lose the excess fluid. Benjamin unwittingly added to the problem by drinking large amounts of water all week, thinking that he needed to stay hydrated. By the time he got out of the ICU several weeks later, he had lost 80 pounds by shedding the excess fluid.

Eventually, he recovered to the point where he had about one-third to one-half of normal heart function. Then in 2008, he had the first of three heart surgeries, after his heart function dropped to about 15-20 percent of normal. He also had a pacemaker/internal defibrillator implanted, and it has saved his life. He tires easily, often takes naps, and works part-time in his own business. While they had planned that Theresa would be the stay-at-home parent, Benjamin has taken on that role. Theresa works three jobs.

Theresa said, "He takes fistfuls of medication every day. Every time he doesn't feel well, he wonders if it's his heart worsening. He worries that the defibrillator will go off while he is driving or while he is watching one of our kids. I worry about the same thing. I start to feel panicked when he doesn't answer the phone before the voicemail picks up."

She said, "If that doctor had just checked his swelling or ordered an x-ray that first day, my husband's heart could have been spared irreparable damage. Every hour counted. He's 38 now and he half-jokes that his goal is to live to see 50. We don't talk about growing old together as it's too painful to admit it probably won't happen. I wonder about life as a widow and how we'll go on if we lose him. I wonder if I'll have to try and explain his death to our kids while they're young, and how to raise them without him if that happens."

Theresa is 34 years old. Their children are now 6, 8, and 10 years old.

The impact on the children is sobering: "We've had to train our kids on how to call 911 if they're home alone with Daddy and something happens to him, and he can't talk or call for help. When he got very sick again a couple of years ago, we had to have them practice what they would say and made sure they could dial on any of our phones and cell phones. That's more reality than a child should have to deal with. The worry never stops. If only that doctor had listened—how very different our lives could have been."

With the benefit of hindsight, Benjamin would change his definition of a "good patient."

Reluctance to challenge the doctor

Research published in 2012 found that patients typically believe that they must not voice disagreement with their doctors. Patients' income, age, race, employment status, health insurance, and education level had no impact on this stance. Even well educated patients with health insurance were reluctant to say anything that might upset their doctors.

Why? They "feared being seen as a difficult patient, . . . thought that disagreement would damage their relationship with their physician, . . . and worried that it might interfere with getting the care that they wanted."[188]

Other researchers, also publishing a new study in 2012, said, "Many participants reported that they did not feel respected or heard because their physician was often authoritarian, rather than authoritative."[189]

A typical patient comment was, "It would feel very uncomfortable if I were in a position where I felt like I were challenging the doctor and essentially challenging his authority. . . . Part of the issue with doctors being gods is if you disagree with him, you're challenging [a] god . . . and you don't want to do that 'cause that's not a very safe thing to do."[190]

That attitude is not surprising; one doctor was quoted saying that many doctors are taught "to think of ourselves as little gods" and view negatively patients who challenge them.[191]

Researchers reported, "Knowing they may need to return at some later time, participants felt they were vulnerable and dependent on the good will of their physicians. Thus, deference to authority instead of genuine partnership appeared to be the participants' mode of working. . . . Participants did not feel they could rely on their physician to help them become aware of and understand treatment options."[192]

One interviewer concluded, "Even the most outspoken and assertive among us may suddenly turn meek when we are sick or vulnerable in a hospital, fearing that our treatment will suffer if we antagonize caregivers."[193]

One hospital CEO said, "It's all too common for patients and family members to remain silent when they suspect something is wrong or improper in their care."[194]

A general lament among health care experts is that individuals don't take a more active role in managing their own health. But they are often discouraged from meaningful involvement—at every step.

Dr. Don Berwick, who once ran the federal agency that oversees Medicare and Medicaid, is fond of saying, "Every process delivers exactly the results it is designed to deliver."[196] If the current system produces patients who are afraid to engage their doctors, then that's exactly what it is designed to do.

> ### SAD BUT TRUE
>
> # 15
>
> Percentage of patients who felt that disagreeing with their doctor could "lead to good outcomes"
>
>
>
> A study involving 1,340 patients, published in 2012 in the *Archives of Internal Medicine*[195]

No voice in choosing which risks to take on

Jonathan had stayed a little later than usual to grade papers. He finished gathering his belongings and stuffed them into his messenger bag. It was after two o'clock on a Friday afternoon, and the community college campus had emptied out for the weekend.

He flung the messenger bag onto his shoulder, and that was the last normal moment he had for a long time. He heard a popping sound in his back and went right to his knees. No one was around and he didn't have his cell phone with him.

"It took me an hour to get 100 yards to my car," he recalled. "It was very, very painful. When I got home, I called my chiropractor and then my GP." They both said that he had strained his back and to come in on Monday—three days later. His doctor prescribed two different painkillers, but "the pain just got worse and worse over the weekend, despite the drugs."

By 2:00 a.m. Monday, "I couldn't stand, sit, lie down, walk—I couldn't do anything—without shrieking in pain."

He called an ambulance and was taken to the local trauma center.

"They said, 'Oh, you just pulled your back out.'"

Jonathan did not agree.

"I objected and said that I wanted an MRI or whatever they needed to do to diagnose it, because I did not simply pull my back out. It took twelve hours for a neurosurgeon to come talk to me, and he really didn't want to do an MRI. I insisted, and finally he agreed, but it took until around 9:00 p.m.—I had been there since about 3:00 a.m.—to get it done. Then the neurosurgeon came to talk to me and told me that I had herniated a disk between L4 and L5 and crushed my spinal canal. He said I needed immediate surgery, or else I could end up paralyzed."

Then the surgeon asked, "Have you taken any aspirin recently?"

"Yes, 81 mg."

"I will have to wait a week to operate, or else you might bleed out."

Jonathan said, "They kept me there for three days on heavy pain medication. Then the neurosurgeon told me that he was discharging me because my health insurance wouldn't pay to keep me in the hospital just waiting for the surgery. I protested, but didn't get anywhere. He said he would give me pain meds to get me through the weekend, and to come back on Monday. This was on Thursday. He gave me five prescriptions for narcotic pain relievers—a fentanyl patch, Dilaudid, OxyContin, Valium, and hydrocodone. I had discharge instructions that said I was supposed to take all of these."

But when his wife went to the drugstore, the pharmacist said, "I can't fill these. If he takes all five of these, he's at risk for respiratory arrest." After phoning the surgeon, he very reluctantly filled them, warning, "Someone will have to stay up with him all night to monitor his breathing."

As predicted, Jonathan started having serious trouble breathing. He cut back to two drugs. "Even so, by Sunday I was psychotic. I couldn't read or write. I could barely speak. I could hardly move. I was completely out of my mind."

When Jonathan returned to the hospital as instructed, he still didn't find the experience smooth sailing; by the time he was settled into his room, it was Monday night. He had successful surgery the next day, eleven days after his injury. He commented, "The worst part of the whole thing was the unsupervised weekend taking five strong narcotics. That was really scary. If my wife hadn't been watching, if I hadn't stopped taking [some of] the drugs, I think I would have stopped breathing."

He concluded, "If a carpenter makes a mistake, a wall isn't plumb or square. If a doctor makes a mistake, somebody dies."

Asking questions about risks and trade-offs

At first glance, the choice between the two alternatives sounds like a toss-up: have surgery right away and possibly die from blood loss, or delay surgery and risk paralysis and narcotic side effects such as death because breathing stops.

Careful analysis, though, leads to a different conclusion. Research suggests that the risk of bleeding out might have been lower than the surgeon implied, and treatments to counteract the effects of aspirin to allow needed surgery to proceed are available. While none of the treatments themselves are free of risk, using them may be less risky than delaying.[198]

But the surgeon did not talk with Jonathan or his wife about which risks Jonathan preferred to take. He did not say anything like, "One person out of one hundred in situations like yours will die of blood loss during surgery. Twenty will end up paralyzed if surgery is delayed. Fifty will stop breathing due to the narcotics, and thirty will have permanent cognitive decline due to drug-induced delirium." (Numbers are for illustration only.)

See the box on the next page for some questions to ask about risks and trade-offs. Even if you can get only partial answers, they may help you figure out which risks you prefer to take on.

How To Consider Risk Trade-Offs

If your doctor proposes waiting to reduce risk, ask:
1. **What risks increase if I wait?**
    (For example, if you are confined to bed, are you at risk for blood clots or pneumonia?)
    a. **How many patients** out of 100 would each affect?
    b. **How serious** are the problems it might cause? (*E.g., a third of people who get blood clots die.*)

2. **What stopgap measures are needed while I wait?**
    (For example, will you need to take narcotic painkillers?)
    Then for each:
    a. What **risks** does this stopgap measure have?
    b. **How many patients** out of 100 would be affected?
    c. **How serious** are the problems it might cause?

3. **If I want to have the treatment right away:**
    a. **What risks are greater** than they'd be if I waited?
    b. **How much greater** are they?
    c. **What steps can be taken** to reduce the risks?

If your doctor rejects an action because of risks:
4. **For each risk, ask:**
    a. **How many patients** out of 100 would that affect?
    b. **How serious** are the problems it might cause?

If your doctor proposes an alternate course:
5. **What are the risks of that treatment?**
    For each risk, ask:
    a. **How many patients** out of 100 would be affected?
    b. **How serious** are the problems it might cause?

Excess and more excess

If doctors almost always made excellent decisions about what tests and treatments to order, patients might have less reason to be concerned about doctors' reluctance to involve them in making care choices. But the evidence doesn't support this optimistic scenario.

For example, your chances of having surgery if you have prostate cancer, back pain, or heart disease are six to ten times greater in some cities than in others.[199] The differences are not due to any significant differences in the patients, their health, their preferences, or their needs. Instead, researchers found that the more specialists and hospital beds per person in a city, the more surgeries performed per person.[201]

> **SAD BUT TRUE**
>
> # 6x-10x
>
> Increased likelihood of having surgery if you live in an area with a high concentration of specialists
>
>
>
> Dr. Don Berwick, who at one time ran the federal organization that oversees Medicare and Medicaid[200]

When researchers compared two matched groups of people age 65-plus who were equally sick, those in the group that got more surgery and other treatment ended up in *worse* health than those in the group that got less care.[202] Like many people, you might assume that "more is better." With health care, it turns out, "more" is often "more likely to kill you."

Besides prescribing treatments that sometimes cause more harm than good, doctors may also order tests that serve no medical purpose. Excessive testing isn't just expensive; it's dangerous.

One study found that many patients are given two CT scans in one session, one without contrast dye and one with dye, an arrangement that experts said was almost never medically necessary. In one hospital, 89 percent of Medicare patients who had CT scans got double scans.[203] CT scans "deliver 100 to 500 times the radiation associated with an ordinary x-ray and now provide three-fourths of Americans' radiation exposure."[204] In fact, 1.5% of all cancers in the U.S. are believed to be caused by CT scans.[205]

Moneymakers

One doctor, who routinely writes for the *New York Times*, noted that a colleague said that he orders at least 10 nuclear stress tests each month to help cover his costs, whether any of his patients actually need such a test or not. "Over-consultation and over-testing have now become facts of the medical profession. The culture in practice is to grab patients and generate volume."[206]

Pointless testing

In 2012, doctors' organizations that represent nine different medical specialties acknowledged that testing often has no impact on treatment plans, regardless of the results.

They recommended significantly reducing the use of specific tests. As one report put it, "The recommendations represent an unusually frank acknowledgment by physicians that many profitable tests and procedures are performed unnecessarily and may harm patients. By some estimates, unnecessary treatment constitutes one-third of medical spending in the United States."[208]

No net benefits

Sometimes, given the choice, you might elect not to treat a condition, or to treat it less invasively (for example, do exercise instead of have surgery), if you knew ahead of time how much the proposed treatment would interfere with your ability to lead the life you want. Consider an example.

A large number of people who have high cholesterol—but haven't had heart attacks or heart disease—would have to take statins (drugs to reduce cholesterol) for one person to benefit. One doctor translated the research results as follows: "What if you put 250 people in a room and told them they would each pay $1,000 a year for a drug they would have to take every day [for years], that many would get diarrhea and muscle pain, and that 249 would have no benefit? . . . How many would take that?"[209]

Many treatments offer a similar profile.

"This treatment is standard practice," your doctor says reassuringly. Or, you might be told, it's the "best practice" or even "the gold standard" for people with your condition. How can you argue with that? What are you implying that you want instead? A "worse practice"?

But calling a treatment the best practice doesn't mean that it is. The Mayo Clinic took a look at all 363 articles that analyzed standard treatments (best practices) in a medical journal over the course of ten years. In 40% of the cases, those current practices were found to be worse than the approaches that doctors used to use—or else doing nothing at all actually got better results than the current approaches.

The studies also concluded that only 38% of the current treatments analyzed were in fact effective. In the remaining 22% of the cases, it wasn't possible to tell if the current treatment was better or worse than the previous one, or even better than no treatment at all.[211]

The "best practices" analyzed included drugs, surgery, medical tests, and so forth.

How can an approach to medical care become the standard when it doesn't actually work or isn't an improvement over an older approach? The Mayo Clinic reports that the practice "gains acceptance largely through vocal support from prominent advocates," even though the evidence in favor of it is often "inadequate, biased, and conflicted." Disturbingly, even when a test or treatment is proven ineffective or even harmful, "removing the contradicted practice often proves challenging."[212]

It's one thing to say that tests and treatments are often overused, or that

> **SAD BUT TRUE**
>
> # 30-50
>
> Percentage of health care tests and treatments that are unnecessary
>
> ❧
>
> Researchers and leaders of many health organizations, based on studies involving millions of patients over three decades[210]

they are often given to patients for whom they aren't a good fit. But the Mayo Clinic study suggested that the problem is even bigger: "A high percentage of all practices [tests and treatments] may ultimately be found to have no net benefits."[213]

When doctors believe that we have the best health care in the world, that side effects are no big deal, and that treatments work for everyone, ordering unneeded tests and treatments may seem harmless.

Power plays

"Doctor knows best" is a dangerous assumption that, loosely speaking, applies to other health care professionals as well as to doctors, meaning that it's rarely the patient who is in control—regardless of the situation.

My mother and I had been waiting in the doctor's examining room for just a few minutes when I wrote her a note: Get doctor now! *I had never before given my mother an order, but she didn't hesitate. Within seconds, the doctor was standing in the doorway, calling over his shoulder to the nurse to arrange an emergency admission to the hospital.*

I had almost stopped breathing. My throat was nearly swollen shut and I couldn't talk. As he rushed me out of the office, the doctor ordered me confined to bed at the hospital, afraid that any movement at all on my part could trigger a coughing attack that would close my throat the rest of the way. I wasn't even allowed to whisper; doing so might similarly irritate and close my throat.

At the hospital, various health care workers bustled in and out of my room. A man pointed to a blue bundle on the nightstand and said, "That's a tracheotomy tray. It's a surgical kit. If your breathing gets any worse, we'll have to perform emergency surgery right here to cut a breathing hole in your neck. You would die before we could get you to an operating room."

I flinched involuntarily.

"Don't worry," he said reassuringly. "Everybody knows you're here. If you have any more trouble breathing than you're having right now, you just press the call button, and someone will come running."

He explained that normally when a patient hits the call button, the nurse calls on the intercom. But since I couldn't talk, someone would always come in person right away, because they wouldn't know if my need was urgent or routine until they got to my room.

After I was settled in, my mother left to go back to work. A couple hours later, I pressed the call button for the first time.

Nobody showed up.

After a short delay, a woman's voice came over the intercom, asking brusquely, "What do you need?"

Of course, I couldn't talk, so I couldn't answer. I wasn't worried, though, because I thought that when she got no response, she would realize, "Oh, this is the girl with the breathing problem!"

Instead, a minute passed and then the voice said sternly, "If you don't say what you need, no one will come."

I froze. I stared at the intercom on the wall in disbelief.

The person on the other end had just cut my lifeline. I was helpless: unable to talk or whisper and tied to the bed by an IV line and by the threat of dying if I got up. I realized in a flash that I could die—at the age of 15, in the hospital, with the surgical tools needed to save my life lying untouched less than two feet away.

You might imagine that the person at the other end of that intercom would think, The children on this floor are very sick. If a patient presses the call button and then doesn't say anything, I'd better see if something is wrong.

But instead her thinking must have been closer to, If a child presses the call button and then doesn't answer me when I speak to her, she must be fooling around, and I won't put up with that. *She seemed determined to call the shots— make sure I knew that I had to follow her rules if I wanted any medical attention.*

I was a well-behaved and scared 15-year-old girl who had never before pressed the call button. The odds that I was deliberately trying to cause trouble were close to zero.

You might think, "Oh, it was just a little oversight. Probably somebody went on break, and the person filling in didn't know about you. They didn't mean anything by it."

On the surface, that's perfectly logical. Dig a little deeper, though, and that excuse breaks down. Unless patients are terminally ill, keeping them breathing should be a very high priority. If it is, then plans for covering lunches and breaks should ensure that patients with breathing problems still get needed attention.

What happened in my case? I had to work hard to avoid panicking—crying and hyperventilating probably would have closed my airway. After the longest twenty minutes of my life, a nurse came tearing into the room, skidding across the linoleum, gasping from the run. My breathing was very labored, but it hadn't gotten much worse; I had called about a routine need.

Once she saw that I was still breathing, she stopped to catch her breath. Then she apologized profusely, promising fervently that such a lapse would not happen again. And it didn't. But once could have been enough to kill me.

Galileo redux

Galileo, an Italian scientist born in the 1500s, was condemned as a heretic by the people in power. Why? He promoted the idea that the earth revolves around the sun, a concept that had the advantage of being true and the disadvantage of being unpopular. Those with power were convinced that the earth—their domain—was the center of the universe. They were outraged when Galileo challenged this conviction.

Patients sometimes run into similar outrage when they try to act on the idea that health care should revolve around them—that it should be designed to meet their needs. But when health care is not designed for the people it is intended to serve, it frequently fails.

11

How did we get here?

People who enter the health care profession typically want to help others. Clearly, nobody goes to work planning to give defective care or wanting to hurt people. Yet the harm patients experience is extensive. Ten beliefs that underlie much of this harm are so ingrained that they are nearly as unremarkable to us as water is to fish:

1. We have the best health care in the world.
2. You'll be fine once the doctor patches you up.
3. Side effects are no big deal.
4. Treatments work for everyone.
5. If you don't get better, it must be your fault.
6. Doctors focus on the important stuff.
7. The diagnosis you get is correct.
8. You don't need to know what's going on.
9. Medical records are for doctors.
10. Doctor knows best.

These assumptions arose in earlier eras when, interestingly, *health care was not about you*. It could get good results without involving you very much. The chart on the next page depicts three eras of health care in the U.S. over roughly the last hundred years,[214] and the text following explains.

Three Eras of Health Care

Era	Causes of Death	What Improves Health	Whose Actions Drive Results	Change in Life Expectancy	What Individuals Need To Do
	Infections	Water Treatment	Public Health Agencies	+44%	**Nothing**
	Injuries Infections	Medical Treatment	Doctors	+13%	**Show Up**
	Chronic Conditions (e.g., heart disease, diabetes)	Prevention	Individuals	?	**Take Charge**

Figure 3

From *When Health Care Hurts* © 2014 by Elizabeth L. Bewley

Three eras of health care

In the first era, people often died of infectious diseases. Health improved when professionals in public health agencies drove efforts to clean up the water supply and improve sewage treatment,[215] leading to a big leap in life expectancy. People born in 1900 on average lived to age 47. People born in 1950 on average are expected to live to age 68.[216] Professionals didn't need to involve each person individually to drive these changes.

In the second era, during the mid-1900s, people still died of *acute conditions* such as infections, injuries, and other problems that arose suddenly. Health improved with *acute interventions*—treatments given once or over a short period of time—such as penicillin, vaccinations,[217] and surgery.

It was the job of doctors like those celebrated in Norman Rockwell paintings to take the actions needed to improve health. Individuals in this era did have to do something: they had to show up. But that's about all. The doctor, who was epitomized by television's fictitious kindly general practitioner Marcus Welby, M.D., did everything else. Average life span rose 9 years.[218]

In this era, the discovery and rapid adoption of one stunningly successful treatment—penicillin—probably spawned most of the dangerous assumptions that underlie health care today. They weren't dangerous when they originally arose; they were reasonably accurate:

- We have the best health care in the world (now that we can treat a major cause of death, infections, with one shot).
- You'll be fine once the doctor patches you up (whereas before an infection like pneumonia led to death a large percentage of the time).
- Side effects are no big deal (when the alternative to this new miracle treatment is a high probability of death).
- Treatments work for everyone (since no bacteria have yet developed resistance to the new miracle drug).
- If you don't get better, it must be your fault (because you must not have bothered to go to the doctor).
- Doctors focus on the important stuff (given that almost nothing could be as important as thwarting a very major cause of death).
- The diagnosis you get is correct (since you get better, which presumably you wouldn't if the diagnosis were wrong).
- You don't need to know what's going on (because the shot will cure

you whether or not you know that your diagnosis is pneumonia and that the drug in the syringe is penicillin).
- Medical records are for doctors (because when you get sick, the doctor gives you a shot and you get better, so your having the records wouldn't change anything).
- Doctor knows best (because doctors are the ones who are delivering the miracle cure).

While these assumptions may have been harmless in the 1950s, it is clear from the first ten chapters of this book that they are harmless no more.

Today we are in the third era. Thanks to the great and continuing successes of the prior eras we now have the "luxury" of dying of chronic diseases, such as diabetes or heart disease. These typically develop slowly and aren't cured, but instead are managed to reduce the harm they cause. Today, 70 percent of people die from chronic conditions.[219]

What counts most in preventing or managing these diseases? It's the actions people take daily regarding diet, exercise, alcohol, tobacco, and stress.[220] People go to the doctor on average three times a year.[221] It's what they do the other 362 days that largely drives their health. Do they go for a bicycle ride or do they play video games? Do they order the small ice cream cone or the triple-decker? Do they fume about their boss or find a constructive way to manage their stress?

When common chronic diseases are the issue, *doctors cannot make good health happen.* They can't snatch the potato chips off your lunch tray. They can't drag you off the couch after dinner to go for a walk instead of watching old *Law & Order* reruns. They're not there to do it. And, unlike the case in the second era, they can't simply give you a shot to make you better.

In this era, rank amateurs—regular people—are the ones who have to take the actions most needed to improve health. But patients and doctors alike are trained to expect the experts to take charge. Patients have been trained to be passive. Doctors have been trained to believe that the grand finale to an illness or injury is the treatment they give. Then the credits roll and the lights come up.

Health care simply hasn't recognized that in this third era, the patient is often the central actor, on stage far more than the doctor. Treatments for chronic illnesses are, by definition, far less likely to resolve your complex medical condition than were the simpler treatments of half a century ago that addressed simpler problems.

Even so, for chronic conditions doctors may try multiple treatments—even dozens or hundreds of them over time—believing that *their* actions must be the ones that can create health. After all, they're the doctors.

The sheer volume of treatments, piled on top of each other over years or decades, creates dramatically more opportunity for errors and complications than may have been the case in prior eras.

Where acute conditions are concerned—a broken hip, holes in the heart, a brain fluid leak, and so forth—today's treatments are often far more invasive and far more of an assault on your body than were treatments available fifty or one hundred years ago, thanks to advances in medical technology.

On one hand, that's great news, because it means that problems that would have led to death a few decades ago are now fixable. On the other hand, it means that chances of complications are exponentially greater.

Managing processes

Historically, doctors had less need than they do today to master "process management," a field created to clarify the purpose of a series of related steps (a "process") and design ways to consistently achieve that purpose.

Today, the difference between managing processes well and badly can mean the difference between life and death for the patient, or between a healthy life and one devastated by disability due to avoidable complications.

Process management was first used most commonly in manufacturing. Some doctors believe that it doesn't apply to health care. After all, a surgeon isn't making hundreds of identical Model T Fords. Each patient is unique, with different symptoms, genetics, medical history, physique, and so forth.

But process management doesn't mean that all patients get the same treatment, even if they have the same condition. Process management means that every detail of every task is deliberately designed to help achieve the *purpose* of the process.

To find the *purpose* of a process, one starts by asking two key questions:

- **Who is intended to benefit from this process?**
- **What do they want from it?**

Attempts to improve a process without understanding its purpose are destined to fail. While some people are tempted to skip the questions because "everybody knows" the answers, the reality might surprise you.

As an example, consider the reporting of medical test results to patients. (Keep in mind the story told in Chapter 9: Shannon wasn't told promptly about medical test results that showed a life-threatening drop in her blood count.)

Suppose that *doctors* are viewed as the primary beneficiaries or customers of the process. They say that reporting normal test results takes up too much of their time. However, they do want to tell people personally about abnormal results.[222] In this case, the purpose of the reporting process might be "to save the doctor's time when results are normal and to have the doctor talk with patients when results are abnormal."

The design might have two features: first, it might or might not include reporting normal results to patients; the customer of the process did not specify. If the process did include reporting these, it would do so without the doctor's involvement and without any urgency—via mail, perhaps.

Second, it would trap abnormal results and send them to the doctor's desk. The customer of the process did not say how quickly patients need to be contacted, so the results might sit indefinitely until the doctor has a chance to call or see the patient.

Suppose, on the other hand, that *patients* are viewed as the primary customers of the process that notifies them of their test results. They say that they want to receive *all* their test results and especially want to get abnormal results right away, so that they can start dealing with any problem.[223] In this case, the purpose might be "to report all test results to patients promptly, in order to minimize stress and reduce failures to treat serious conditions caused by delays or failures in getting test results to patients."

The design might include a way to report all test results to patients the same day they are first available, or shortly thereafter. This might be done via electronic notification (with security features to protect privacy) or perhaps via phone calls from one of the doctor's staff.

If staff members called with abnormal results, they could immediately schedule patients to see the doctor. If the notification were electronic, alerts could be built in so that patients with seriously abnormal results who did not call promptly to make an appointment would be called by a member of the office staff.[224]

The differences in the solutions arise from differences in who the customers of the process are considered to be and their different needs.

Consider the story in Chapter 8 about Charles, who did not remember anything the doctor told him to do. The suggestions offered to improve his recall follow logically from answers to the questions about who the customer of the office visit is and what he needs from it.

For doctors to deliver optimal care, it's important for them to understand the concept of process management and to carefully design and run processes in their practices that will achieve the purposes identified. These processes include everything from how patients schedule appointments to how the doctor performs surgery.

Similarly, hospitals need to manage processes, and doing so means working with doctors to coordinate care so that patients get the best results.

Many steps

To make the concept of process management more concrete, an example of a process and ways in which it can fail is given here. In this example, suppose that your knee hurts. You are the customer of the process, and the purpose of the process is to enable you to use your knee as you did before, without pain. The process of getting care may involve a dozen steps or more:

1. You realize that something is wrong.
2. You decide you need medical care.
3. You decide where to get it (emergency room, doctor's office, or other location).
4. Unless it is an emergency, you call to make an appointment.
5. You make arrangements to keep the appointment. For example, you change your work schedule or ask someone to watch your children.
6. You may try to reduce the pain, perhaps by taking pain relievers.
7. You go to the doctor's office.
8. A nurse or medical assistant asks questions and takes notes.
9. The doctor examines you, makes notes, and gives instructions.
10. You go to a drug store to fill a prescription, a medical supply house to buy a knee brace, and a sporting goods store to get ankle weights.
11. You change your routine based on the doctor's instructions. For example, you take medicine, do leg exercises, and so forth.
12. After some time, you realize that you feel better—or that you don't. If you don't, you start the process all over again.[225]

Notice that you're the one who has to take most of the steps. The doctor doesn't. You're the key actor in executing this process.[226]

SAD BUT TRUE

54

Percentage of the time that a process with 12 steps will work right if each step is done correctly 95 percent of the time

✿

The equation is 12 instances of .95 multiplied together

Many things can go wrong with even a simple care process. Examples of typical gaps on the patient's side follow. (Assume that the diagnoses and doctor's advice are valid.)

First, actions you take at home may mask symptoms or worsen your condition. For example, a pain killer may also reduce fever, leading the doctor to assume that you don't have an infection when you do. Doctors typically don't ask what you did to treat the problem before the office visit.

Second, you might mistakenly assume that the nurse or medical assistant passed on to the doctor everything you just said, so you might omit important information when the doctor walks in, assuming that it's already in your chart.

Third, the doctor and the patient may not understand each other. For example, when my husband was three years old, he complained that his foot hurt. The doctor examined his foot and said it was fine. Later, it became clear that the boy had a broken leg—he had simply described the location of the pain imprecisely.

Fourth, patients typically forget the instructions they are given.[227]

Fifth, patients may not understand instructions.

Sixth, patients may not follow advice. One study found that almost half of us say that we have ignored a doctor's advice.[228]

Seventh, patients may not realize that they have questions until they get home or even until several days have passed.

For example, I was once given the instruction: "Don't lift anything over five pounds." When I pulled a file out of a tightly packed desk drawer, I did not think until later that while the file itself weighed only a few ounces, I had to exert a lot of force to tug it free. Was that the same as lifting something that weighed over five pounds? Was it okay to pick up my big dictionary? I found out later that it weighed seven pounds. The doctor gave a simple instruction. But it wasn't at all clear to me once I left his office.

If told to take medicine an hour before meals, what happens if you have a snack right before that? Does the instruction mean to take the drug on an empty stomach? What counts as an empty stomach? Is it better to skip the dose or go ahead and take it on a stomach full of chips and dip?

If the medical advice matters, then it is in the details like these that health care either succeeds or fails. If people do not know and cannot get the right answers, they may be acting at cross-purposes to the doctor.

An eighth gap is that patients may understand the instructions but not why they matter. If they don't understand their medical conditions and have little say in treatment plans, they may not take them seriously.

> **SAD BUT TRUE**
>
> # 9 in 10
>
> Adults who "have difficulty following routine medical advice, largely because it's often incomprehensible to average people"
>
>
>
> The Centers for Disease Control and Prevention, quoted in the *Wall Street Journal*[29]

The above are simply a few examples of gaps; hundreds or thousands more exist. And most health care is much more complex than the above example of a basic office visit and its aftermath, and thus much more likely to fail. When a single test is ordered, more than a dozen steps may be added:

1. The doctor figures out the right test to order.
2. The doctor's office staff gets insurance authorization, if necessary.
3. The doctor talks with the individual to gain agreement for the test.
4. The individual schedules the test and arranges to be available for it.
5. The individual follows pretest instructions.
6. The individual shows up at the test site.
7. The test site collects the specimen or conducts the test correctly.
8. The analyst performs the analysis correctly. (For instance, the lab work is done right or the x-ray is interpreted accurately.)
9. The analyst notes the results correctly with the right patient's name.
10. The test site reports the results to the doctor.

11. The doctor receives and reads the report.
12. The doctor interprets the results appropriately.
13. The doctor notifies the individual of the results (one hopes).
14. The doctor recommends further testing or treatment if needed.

Processes often involve hand-offs from one person to another. Notice above how many different people have to act: the doctor, the doctor's staff, an insurance company employee, test site employees, analysts, and the patient.

It is easy for whole processes to fail due to a small mistake in any step. For example, suppose that the doctor accidentally checks the wrong box on the form to order a blood test. The individual can show up for the test. The lab can perform it correctly and report accurately. The patient can be told, "Your blood test was normal." In fact, she could have a serious problem that the correct test would have revealed.

The purpose of health care

You might be surprised to hear that there isn't a standard, agreed-upon answer to the question, "What is the purpose of health care?" If you ask a doctor, you might hear: "To diagnose and treat disease."[230]

Public policy experts might say: "To improve population health," which means using the available money to get the best health outcomes for the greatest number of people for the longest period of time. For instance, spending money to clean up the water supply and create better sewage treatment systems was and continues to be one of the best ways to improve population health.

Having read the previous chapters, you might conclude that the actual purpose of the health care system today is *to deliver tests and treatments.* The health care system certainly does that. For example, each year there are 130 million trips to emergency rooms, 101 million hospital outpatient visits, and 37 million hospital admissions.[231]

What happens if you back up a step to ask who the primary beneficiaries (or customers) of health care are? You might answer, "the people who need/ receive care."[232]

Then consider the second process design question: what do they want (from health care)? Most people don't want to be patients; having a medical problem that requires dealing with the health care system is a huge and unwelcome disruption. What they want is to get back to their normal lives.

Putting together those two answers, one could conclude that health care's purpose should be *to enable people to lead the lives they want.*

Of course, health care can't solve every medical problem, and other resources are needed for people to lead the lives they want. That said, many people might conclude that it is not good enough for health care to act as if its purpose is simply *to deliver tests and treatments.*

Consider what Dr. Don Berwick, a proponent of individual-centric health care, had to say: "I have come to believe that we—patients, families, clinicians, and the health care system as a whole—would all be far better off if we professionals recalibrated our work such that we behaved with patients and families not as hosts in the care system, but as guests in their lives."[233]

12

When health care is about you

Your life will improve when health care's purpose becomes *to enable people to lead the lives they want.*

Making it possible to do the things that matter to you

Sarah, 47, is a single mother with two children in college. Her ad agency job involves using a computer all day, and she developed carpal tunnel syndrome in both wrists.

After simpler treatments failed to provide any relief, she had surgery on one wrist. The plan was to have surgery on the other wrist once she recovered. Events didn't work out as planned. A week after the operation, she saw the surgeon for a check-up. The surgeon looked at her arm with alarm.

"On a scale of one to ten," he asked, "how much does it hurt? 'Ten' is the worst pain you can imagine."

"About fifty," Sarah promptly replied.

"I will meet you at the hospital," the surgeon said, picking up his jacket.

Sarah had contracted necrotizing fasciitis—a fast-moving infection that is often fatal. After multiple operations and one crisis after another, her doctors said that she was going to die. All her family members flew in from around the country and took up a vigil at the hospital. Miraculously, she survived. However, she lost almost all the use of one arm—despite more than two dozen operations.

After all the surgery, Sarah did not get much out of the two or three home visits from an occupational therapist. She has been in physical therapy for over a year now. They routinely measure how far she can bend her fingers, to see if she is improving. However, when Sarah recently talked about her situation, she didn't say things like, "I wish I could bend my fingers another 20 degrees."

She said, "I love to cook. But it takes me three times as long now. It's nearly impossible to chop vegetables with one hand, so I don't cook." She said, "I love to read. But I can't hold the book and turn the pages, so I don't read any more." She said, "It's embarrassing when I eat in a restaurant. I have to ask someone else to cut my meat for me."

Sarah's inability to handle so many everyday tasks robbed her of much of her joy in life. She found it hard to plan and follow through on plans. She became depressed, mourning the loss of her former life and the things she could do when she had two working arms. No one told her that there were simple fixes that could address the obstacles that so disheartened her. Yet such solutions abound.

A food processor with a wide mouth can chop vegetables. A rocker knife makes it possible to cut meat one-handed. Clever storage canisters that seal tightly and yet open easily with one hand are now on the market. Non-slip mats can be placed under bowls or cutting boards to keep them from moving. Book holders make it possible to enjoy reading. There is even a book called One-Handed in a Two-Handed World *that offers hundreds of practical solutions. (The book is spiral-bound, making it easy to read one-handed.)*

Once an acquaintance told her about these products, Sarah's life changed.

"I put the non-skid mat on the counter and put a cutting board on it. That book said to use a meat cleaver to chop vegetables. I had a meat cleaver, but it never would have occurred to me to use it for vegetables. I tried it, and the cutting board didn't move, and the meat cleaver worked like a charm. I can't believe it!"

The joy in her voice was evident as she said, "I see all sorts of possibilities that I thought were gone forever!"

The health care system spent hundreds of thousands of dollars treating Sarah—and still failed her. It is common for patients to be left almost entirely on their own to figure out—or to not figure out—how to function within the limits of their disabilities.

For example, people who break a bone may spend six or eight miserable weeks in a cast. Within days, they may start to feel subhuman because bathing seems too hard, since the cast has to be kept dry. It turns out that medical supply houses offer a variety of effective waterproof covers for casts.

How To Address Functional Limitations

1. **Explain problems to your doctor in terms of what they prevent you from doing.**
    For example:
    a. Instead of, "My hands hurt," try saying, "I can't play the piano anymore because of pain in my hands.
    b. Instead of, "My hearing isn't that great," try saying, "I can't talk with my sister in Ohio anymore because I can't hear her on the telephone."

2. **Ask your doctor for practical, specific solutions.**

3. **If offered occupational therapy:**
    a. **Identify activities** you care most about doing.
    b. **List** the activities in order of importance.
    c. **Make a plan** with the therapist with goals and time-lines for successfully managing each.

4. **Find assistive devices designed to help.**
    a. **Ask** your occupational therapist.
    b. **Search the internet** for devices for particular body parts or functions, such as "assistive devices-cooking."

They allow people to shower without worrying about getting their casts wet. But often no one tells patients about this solution.

Sarah's story illustrates that health care often doesn't act as if its goal is *to enable people to lead the lives they want*. If that becomes its goal, what will change?

The big change: regarding patients with respect

Understood deeply, this simple idea will shake the foundations of health care. Examples of aspects of health care that will change include: design of care, priorities for research, physician education, and restrictions that insurers place on paying for treatments.

A transforming idea: designing care to meet patients' needs

I have long proposed that health care be designed *to enable people to lead the lives they want*. The *New England Journal of Medicine* recently proposed a similar concept. It started by acknowledging, "So far, assessments of quality of care and health outcomes have not incorporated patient-centeredness."[234] Think about that for a moment. It means that conclusions about how good health care is haven't taken into account what the patient thinks.

The article suggested that patients may have goals such as avoiding falls, being able to get to the bathroom without assistance, and staying in touch with family via the internet. On the other hand, a patient may not consider it a high priority to walk without a walker or to eliminate a mild tremor.

Designing care to meet the patient's goals allows a greater focus, typically less treatment, more interest on the patient's part in participating in care, and often better results. The biggest obstacle is that health care is focused on managing diseases, "rather than asking what patients want."[235]

The *Wall Street Journal* reported on a similar concept: "A focus on quality of life helps medical providers see the big picture—and makes for healthier, happier patients." It terms this shift "the simple idea that is transforming health care." It is built around one question that doctors are encouraged to ask patients: "How is your health affecting your quality of life?"

"The logic is simple," as people can more easily relate to goals such as "being able to do more at work or keep up with their kids, instead of focusing only on comparatively abstract targets like blood-sugar levels."[236]

Similarly, the *New England Journal of Medicine* recently observed,

"Whereas doctors and hospitals focus on producing health care, what people really want is health."[237] I would go one step further and say that what people really want is to be able to do the things that being healthy permits; health by itself isn't the end goal.

Researching how to get better results for you with less risk

Seven key areas include: improving diagnostic accuracy, assessing individuals' real-life risks, managing co-morbidities (multiple diseases in the same person), matching patients to treatments, communicating to reduce stress, eliciting behavior change, and finding the secrets of placebo responders.

Research Topic #1: Improving diagnostic accuracy

When health care is patient-centered, the speed and accuracy of diagnosis will improve. While it can be almost impossible to reach a diagnosis in some cases, focused efforts could eliminate the vast majority of today's errors and lengthy delays:

- Choose a group of patients whose medical records are readily available electronically.
- Identify common conditions that are often misdiagnosed.
- For patients diagnosed with those conditions, find in their medical records the date when each first reported relevant symptoms.
- Note the date when each was first given an accurate diagnosis.
- Calculate the time from first report of symptoms to accurate diagnosis for each patient.
- Analyze the records to identify the false starts and missteps that created delays and errors.
- Create specific solutions for each type of delay and error, using standard process improvement methods.

Is such research practical? Yes. Consider the perspective offered to me by a senior executive with an organization that provides health care for nine million people.

He pointed out that among those enrollees are almost certainly half a million with any major chronic condition one might name. The organization can draw on its electronic records of people with diabetes, heart disease, asthma, and so forth to see the results they actually get from different reputable treatments. Records like these could almost certainly be used for the research described above to improve diagnostic speed and accuracy.

Research Topic #2: Assessing individuals' real-life risks

Health risks that are likely to interfere with individuals' ability to lead the lives they want may not "fit into the disease/specialist model of health care, which tends to focus on things like heart attacks and strokes."[238]

For instance, "for a 75-year-old with high blood pressure, the risk of death or serious disability resulting from a fall is just as high as the risk of death or serious disability caused by a stroke."[239] Research shows that it's possible to tell who is at risk for falls and to make changes to reduce the risk, but this issue is often overlooked.

Similarly, malnutrition is a commonly overlooked and serious risk in the elderly: they may have trouble driving, shopping for groceries, preparing meals, remembering to eat, and so forth.

Research will provide insight into the most effective ways to assess individuals' real health risks and go on to provide guidance about how to forestall or address the most serious ones.

Research Topic #3: Managing co-morbidities (multiple diseases)

As Robert discovered when diabetes and an eye disease contributed to his going blind when he took a blood thinner (Chapter 2), little attention has gone into how to treat people who have more than one medical condition.

The *New England Journal of Medicine* reported, "Almost 3 in 4 individuals aged 65 years and older have multiple chronic conditions, as do 1 in 4 adults younger than 65 years who receive health care. Adults with multiple chronic conditions are the major users of health care services at all adult ages, and account for more than two-thirds of health care spending."[240]

Yet, "The default position is to treat complicated patients as collections of malfunctioning body parts rather than as whole human beings."[241] One expert noted, "You go to a primary care doctor, and then you see four or five specialists, none of whom really talk to each other. . . . It is totally uncoordinated. It's chaotic. It serves pieces of people, not whole people."[242]

Good news in this arena is that geriatrics specialists recently published "Guiding Principles for the Care of Older Adults with Multimorbidity,"[243] an excellent step. They have also prepared a tip sheet for patients called "Living with Multiple Health Problems: What Older Adults Should Know," available at the Foundation for Health in Aging at http://www.healthinaging.org/resources/resource:living-with-multiple-health-problems-what-older-adults-should-know/.

Further research in this area will almost certainly be funded by non-business organizations, for two reasons. First, it will not focus on a particular drug or medical device. Second, the government has the biggest incentive to act, because Medicare pays most of the costs of care for the elderly, who are the ones most likely to have multiple health problems.

Research Topic #4: Matching patients to treatments

As discussed in Chapters 3 and 4, treatments don't work for everyone, and side effects and complications are common. Health, quality of care, and costs will all dramatically improve when it is possible to tell ahead of time who is likely to benefit from a specific treatment. Any given treatment will be provided to only about one-fourth as many people as it is today—but those people will get significant benefits from it.

Genomics will certainly provide part of the solution. Another will come by analyzing the medical records of millions of people to find out the characteristics of those whose health improved after a specific treatment, compared to those whose health stayed the same or worsened.

Research Topic #5: Communicating to reduce stress

The experience of care will improve when communication improves. As an example, communication will help reduce the uncertainty and stress patients often feel. The health care system traditionally creates high stress levels for people in almost all steps in the process of health care—getting a diagnosis, undergoing treatment, and so forth.

An example of relevant research involves informing people about waiting times in an ER. One study reported, "Patients who waited more than four hours to see a doctor, but felt well-informed about the delay, scored more than twice as high on overall satisfaction as those who waited just an hour but considered communication to be 'very poor.'"[244] In other words, *knowing* what is happening dramatically improves people's experience, even if what is happening isn't ideal.

As another example, research will figure out what hospitalized patients most need to know about how care in the hospital works, to reduce their stress. Perhaps what they most need to know is how long they can expect to wait for help once they press the call button and what to do if they need help faster. Perhaps what they most need to know is who is in charge of their care and when/how often they can expect to see that professional. And so forth.

Research Topic #6: Eliciting behavior change

Research will address what it takes for people to make long-lasting changes in their behavior and specify how doctors and other health care professionals can successfully foster such changes. As an example, one need is to find vivid ways to help people genuinely understand the health issues they face.

People who prepare information for executives know that it's critical to provide a clear picture of the issues so that they can make informed decisions, even though they aren't the experts in every single topic. It is—or should be—the job of the health care system to make it very clear to the people it serves the consequences of following different courses of action.

Smokers who were told their "lung age" stopped smoking at twice the rate of those who were simply told their results on a breathing test. Interestingly, even if people were told that their lung age was the same as their chronological age, they stopped smoking at twice the rate of the people who weren't told their lung age.[245]

With that success in mind, imagine a computer model that does the equivalent of time-lapse photography into the future regarding health conditions and behaviors. Individuals will identify from an extensive drop-down menu activities that they care most about being able to do. These might include working, taking care of their children, managing their finances, traveling, and so forth.

Then they will add three other kinds of information: their current health status, including any chronic conditions such as diabetes; their behaviors related to diet, exercise, alcohol, tobacco, and stress; and treatments they are getting. For instance, individuals will select different behaviors from extensive choices to describe their usual routines ("I eat salads every day," or "I live on cheeseburgers and fries," for example.)

Then the computer model will fast-forward 10 or 20 years and calculate the odds that they'll still be able to do each of the things they care about. For example, the model might report: "The probability that you will still be able to drive ten years from now is 67 percent." People will be able to change the treatments and behaviors they've selected to see how the odds change.

Providing people with these projections will be one way to help them understand the significance—in terms that matter to them—of any health issues they have and the consequences of their choices.[246]

Research will also figure out how to communicate in ways likely to engage and energize patients—as opposed to discouraging and deflating them. For example, compare how two different doctors responded to a patient's report of symptoms the doctors couldn't explain:

- "That's ridiculous! That didn't happen!"
- "I've never run across that. But anything is possible. I learn new things from my patients every day."[247]

The second response is clearly more likely to keep the patient engaged. It came from a doctor at the Mayo Clinic, where they focus on treating patients with respect.[248]

Research Topic #7: Finding the secrets of placebo responders

Some people experience improved health through mechanisms that defy current understanding.

For example, in one study, a number of hotel housekeepers were told that their daily work—changing bed sheets and cleaning bathrooms—was a healthy workout. Within four weeks, they lost an average of two pounds and saw modest improvements in their blood pressure, body fat, and BMI (Body Mass Index, a common measure of fitness).

Housekeepers in the control group weren't told anything about their work contributing to their health. Their health measures were unchanged after four weeks.[249]

As another example, in studies of new drugs, some people improve even though they are in the group not given the active drug ingredient. Listen to how these people are described: "They are the people who ruin clinical trials for drug companies: placebo responders, who get better on sugar pills. Drug makers want to get rid of them [exclude them from clinical trials]."[250]

Consider that perspective: these people *ruin* health care research by getting better. What would happen if patients were accorded more respect—if their interest in the benefits that good health offers were the top priority?

The story of Alexander Fleming offers some hints. Researchers have long performed experiments that involved growing organisms in the lab. They were sometimes disheartened when their experiments were ruined by an unknown fungus that killed off the organisms they were trying to grow. In exasperation, they would toss the ruined experiments into the trash.

In 1928, Alexander Fleming investigated the mold that killed one of his cultures—and thus discovered penicillin.[251] (It took more than a decade to develop an effective version that could be manufactured on a large scale.)[252]

In the future when health care is about you, instead of being metaphorically tossed in the trash for ruining the experiments, placebo responders will be studied to discover how they get better without heavy-duty drugs or surgery. They will be revered rather than reviled.

One classic set of research studies in a different field offers a fascinating glimpse into the possibilities. Starting in 1924, researchers at the Western Electric Hawthorne Works factory created a series of experiments to see if worker productivity could be increased with changes in lighting levels.

Unexpectedly, productivity rose both when lighting levels were raised and when they were lowered—and then dropped when the study ended. This result was later termed the Hawthorne effect. One interpretation of the facts is that it was the attention being paid to the workers that made the difference, rather than the specific changes introduced.[253]

Some researchers have speculated that the placebo effect typically seen in studies of drugs, surgery, and other treatments may be in part the result of similar attention. Researchers necessarily show an interest in the people in the studies. They ask them questions, take notes, measure and test various markers of health, and otherwise indicate that the presence and well-being of the study participants are important. Could it be that a few hours of sincere attention could result in health improvements similar to those that are often elusive even with expensive drugs and surgery? What other mechanisms might account for some part of the placebo response?

When health care is truly about you, studying placebo responders will be a major research priority. It may result in great benefits to you at a fraction of today's risks and cost. Since the research probably will not lead to sales of drugs or medical devices, it will be run by non-business organizations such as the National Institutes of Health.

Training doctors

What medical education generally *produces* is doctors who specialize in fields such as heart disease or joint problems, are trained by treating people primarily in hospitals, and expect to call the shots. What the health care system *needs* is more doctors who care for the whole person, emphasize prevention, and support people so they can successfully take charge of their own health and health care.[254]

Either the way in which doctors are created will change, or other health care professionals will be created to oversee patient care to address the above critical needs. If doctors want to continue to play a leading role, three aspects of medical training will change: content of class work, content of hands-on training, and selection of students (future doctors).

First, classroom content will change[255] to add or emphasize key topics:

Understanding the health care landscape
- Purpose of health care: *to enable people to lead the lives they want.*
- Health drivers: 40 percent behavior, 30 percent genetics, and so forth.
- Patient demographics: percentage of hospital patients who are age 65-plus, have multiple problems, die of chronic conditions, etc.
- Magnitude of unintended consequences in health care: number of people harmed by side effects and complications of care annually; percentage of all deaths caused by health care.
- Percentages of patients helped vs. harmed by each of the hundred highest-volume treatments delivered today.
- Magnitude of/reasons for diagnostic errors, including false positives.

Respecting the patient
- Individual-centric health care: supporting people who take charge of their own health and health care.
- Situational leadership: supporting patients who want to make all the major decisions, those who don't, and those in between.
- Respect and disrespect in interactions with patients: what they look like and how they affect the outcomes of care.

Designing care to get intended results
- Process management: how to clarify who is intended to benefit from a process and what they want from it; how to connect the dots to get the desired outcomes.

- Care coordination: why it is needed and the doctor's role.
- Prevention and management of chronic conditions.
- Psychology of patient behavior and how to help people change.

Managing common, complex care situations
- Care for people with multiple health issues: setting priorities for treatment, watching for drug interactions, and so forth.[256]
- Geriatrics (issues unique to the care of the elderly),[257] which among many other topics includes the philosophy of "slow medicine," which involves thoughtfully planning for inevitable crises and avoiding heedlessly piling on multiple high-tech, aggressive, invasive treatments unlikely to help.[258]

In addition to changing the content of classroom education, a second change in physician education is that hands-on training for medical students will be modified to shift some training time from hospital settings to primary care, nursing homes, and hospice.

Third, a change in admission profiles will produce more doctors whose perspectives and interests fit better with the most common medical needs people have today. Health care still needs brain surgeons—I can attest to that. However, the ratio of specialists to generalists is skewed today.

Insurers insisting that you have a say

It's common to hear stories about seemingly arbitrary limits that health insurers place on what treatments they will pay for. A more cost-effective alternative that treats patients with more respect is *to mandate that patients be included in decisions about what is going to be done to them.*

One study found that people had a real say in treatment choices only 9 percent of the time.[259] When given meaningful information about different treatment options—and a voice—"they tend to choose less-invasive and less-expensive treatments than they would have otherwise received."[260]

Research shows that doctors often don't mention risks of tests or treatments.[261] The new mandate will require that you be alerted to both risks and benefits of each major test and treatment proposed and to the risks and benefits of alternatives, including foregoing a test or treatment entirely.

Useful decision aids (documents that explain treatment characteristics and alternatives) have the following characteristics:

- They are unbiased.
- They are written in language that most people can understand.[262]
- They make it easy to compare options.
- They describe expected results in terms patients care about. (For example, it is helpful to say, "The patient will be able to walk around the block without pain," rather than saying only, "The patellar tendon will be debrided.")

Decision aids can help people play an active role in their own care, understand their choices, have realistic expectations, and choose care consistent with their priorities and values.

Doctors sometimes worry that patients will make bad decisions if given choices. If people do, it probably means either that the information provided isn't clear—or that they have priorities and concerns that lead them to a conclusion different from the doctor's. Typically, no one asks them why they've made a given choice. If they were regarded with more respect, they would be asked.

13

What will it take to fix health care?

Health care in the United States accidentally injures or kills staggeringly large numbers of people each year. Most of these deaths are avoidable, using approaches to process management that are proven to be successful. Yet the problems persist. The underlying cause is a systemic lack of respect for patients on the part of the health care system, and the fix proposed follows from this fact.

Poor results from health care

Annual deaths from health care in the U.S. include:

Deaths from selected health care causes

Deaths from blood clots related to hospital care	190,000
Deaths from hospital-acquired infections	75,000
Deaths from medical errors in hospitals	200,000
Deaths from adverse drug events, all locations	305,000
Gross deaths from selected health care causes	**770,000**
Less estimated double counts	(38,000)
Net deaths from selected health care causes	**732,000**[263]

Problems with care are the direct cause of 732,000 deaths a year. That's equivalent to (accidentally) killing off every man, woman, and child in the cities of Boston and Cambridge, Massachusetts.[264] Every year.

By way of comparison, consider how the country responds to deaths of much smaller numbers of people. For example, in 2014, General Motors faced a congressional investigation and criminal charges related to the deaths of 13 people over the course of a decade from a cause that they allegedly knew about but did not address in a timely manner.

Issues such as oil spills, cruise ship or ferry accidents, plane crashes, shootings in schools, mine cave-ins, and so forth—with injuries or deaths ranging from a handful to a few hundred—get extensive news coverage, investigations, and demands for radical changes in operating procedures, just as the GM auto problem did.

In the same decade as the GM issue, health care was the direct and primary cause of death for about 7.3 million people in the United States.

Where's the outrage? Where's the congressional inquiry? Where's the demand for—and commitment to—change?

A social revolution

Fixing health care will take a social revolution on the order of the one that freed the slaves or the one that gave women the vote. Before those revolutions, people with power made critical decisions for—and had control over what happened to—those two underclasses: women and slaves.

One of their justifications was the dubious notion that women and slaves didn't have the mental capacity or interest in complex matters necessary to be in charge of their own lives. Women and slaves were severely discounted and their concerns marginalized.

Individuals—patients—are in a very similar situation today. This revolution will make it unacceptable for the health care system to treat patients as second-class citizens whose intelligence, priorities, values, and needs can be safely ignored.

One could spend the next hundred years trying to fix each failure to treat individuals as if their priorities and their lives counted. For example, a campaign could be launched to dim the lights at night in ICUs to help stave off delirium. The campaign that's been running *for over 165 years* to try to get doctors to wash their hands could be continued. And so forth.

But time is running out. Too many people are dying, and the health care system is on the verge of collapsing under its own weight.

The problem with health care is not that it hurts people nearly as often as it helps them. The problem with health care is not that it is the direct cause of 29 percent of the deaths in this country. *The problem with health care is that patients are viewed with so little regard that exposing them to grave harm on a large scale is not seen as a crisis that warrants immediate action.*

How else can you account for the fact that good people in charge dismiss as *unimportant* the fact that the environment they create in ICUs literally and unnecessarily drives two-thirds of patients insane, with grave long-term consequences for a significant portion of them?[265] (See Chapter 2.) The only explanation for the thousands of issues like this in health care is that people who seek help from the health care system are as discounted and marginalized as women and slaves in this country once were.

Consider other social revolutions. Forty years ago people rarely wore seat belts, drunk driving was common, and cigarette smoke formed a haze in public buildings. Today most people wear seat belts, drunk driving is viewed as irresponsible, and more and more sites are smoke-free.

While some of the mechanisms differed, change efforts in all three cases were built on the same foundation: the new, radical belief that bad outcomes in these areas were not unavoidable, but were instead the direct result of choices people were making.

The same is true in health care. Hospital-acquired infections, blood clots, bedsores, and delirium are not acts of God. Neither are misdiagnosis, excessive testing and treatment, and drug dosing mistakes. These devastating errors that ruin or prematurely end patients' lives are all largely the results of choices made by people involved in providing health care. They have the option of making other choices.

What's required is a social revolution to change unspoken beliefs and attitudes, so that you are treated with respect.

Conclusion

Billboards advertise miracles in treating heart attacks and cancer. By reading *When Health Care Hurts*, you've educated yourself about "the other half" of the story—the part that the health care system doesn't advertise.

Fresh from reading about horrific failures in health care, it's important to remember that the first half does exist—doctors, nurses, hospitals, and all the other players in health care often do a spectacular job taking care of people, improving and saving lives as a result.

This story isn't about good guys and bad guys. It's about broken processes founded on ten dangerous assumptions. With the perspective you've gained by reading this book, you are in a much better position to understand how to get the great benefits that health care can offer, while reducing the odds of having your care—and your life—derailed by common assumptions that can result in harm to you.

I wish you all the best in your quest for health—and for health care that *enables you to lead the life you want.*

Appendix A

Why won't the usual solutions work?

The real issues that patients face

Twelve proposed solutions to the health care crisis are commonly discussed by lawmakers and policymakers. Many are excellent ideas, but all are likely to fail unless they are placed into this larger context: health care's focus needs to shift so that it is genuinely about you, with its goal being *to enable people to lead the lives they want*. As you read about each of the commonly proposed solutions, ask yourself whether it would have made any difference for people whose stories are told in this book:

- Bob, when he was almost killed by a drug mix-up in the hospital as he awaited heart surgery
- Christine, who died of an infection she got in the hospital
- Louise, who nearly died due to a blood clot after surgery
- Mildred, who never went home again as a result of hospital delirium
- Robert, whose care left him blind—when he was already deaf
- Linda, who was permanently disabled by a fall in the shower when the home health agency neglected to take proper precautions
- Alesandra, who got sicker when each new side effect was treated with a new drug
- Lawrence, whose liver nearly failed due to a drug side effect

- Rebecca, who became suicidal when given drugs for depression
- Hannah, who nearly died from the formulas her doctor insisted she be given
- Don, who still suffers greatly from bedsores he got in the hospital ten years ago
- Stacy, whose bladder problem was assumed to be all in her head
- Amber, whose brain infection was misdiagnosed as diabetes
- Michelle, when a mistake nearly led to surgery on the wrong leg
- Tom, who was taken for a medical test ordered for someone else
- Jack, who didn't know what to expect as he recovered from colon surgery
- Shannon, who didn't get her test results showing a dangerously low blood count
- Janice, whose doctor's records showed plans for gall bladder surgery instead of plans for a lap pool
- Terry, whose PTSD was caused by drugs she had explicitly refused
- Benjamin, whose doctor's lack of urgency in addressing his symptoms led to severe heart failure
- Jonathan, whose surgeon ignored the risks of delaying surgery

Twelve commonly proposed fixes

- UNIVERSAL COVERAGE (Everyone has health insurance)
- SINGLE PAYER (The government pays for health care for everyone)
- REGULATION (Restrictions are set on the relationships between companies that make health products and the doctors and hospitals that use them)
- COST CONTROLS (Medicare, the federal health program for the elderly and disabled, cuts the prices it pays)
- HEALTH INFORMATION TECHNOLOGY (HIT) (Through electronic medical records and artificial intelligence programs, care is managed better)
- COMPARATIVE EFFECTIVENESS (An impartial organization researches and reports which treatments work better than others)
- TRANSPARENCY (Information about quality and cost is easy to get)
- CONSUMER-DIRECTED HEALTH PLANS (CDHP) (People shop carefully for health care because of financial incentives)

- PAY FOR PERFORMANCE (P4P) (Doctors are paid more if they deliver better care and less if they deliver worse care)
- FOCUSED CARE (Care providers are organized according to treatment or disease, and they compete on delivering the best outcomes for those)
- ACCOUNTABLE CARE ORGANIZATIONS (Multiple doctors and one or more hospitals work together to manage cost and quality for a specified group of people)
- MEDICAL HOMES (Primary care doctors coordinate all care needed for their patients)

Proposals to fix health care remind me of the old fable in which blind men are asked to describe an elephant. One touches its leg and says, "The elephant is like a tree trunk." The second touches its belly and says, "The elephant is like a wall." The third touches its ear and says, "The elephant is like a piece of cloth." The fourth grabs its tail and says, "The elephant is like a rope."[266]

They were all correct, but they missed the larger picture. Similarly, proposals to fix health care are typically insightful, but they all miss the larger picture. A number of them create essential groundwork, but collectively they are not sufficient to move the dial.[267]

Universal Coverage

The premise:
Everyone should have health insurance. It may come from an employer or the government or be purchased privately. Various subsidies and safety nets are suggested to make coverage available for people who couldn't otherwise afford it.

The limitations:
- The same quality issues that the health care system has today would affect more people. Fewer people would die due to under treatment—but more would die due to medical errors and other side effects and complications.[268]
- Doctors and nurses don't have time to treat more people.
- All but one or two of the people whose stories are told here had health insurance, which did not prevent horrific problems.

Single Payer

The premise:
The United States could save $128 billion a year, by one estimate,[269] if we did what many other developed countries do and had our government pay for health care for all.

The limitations:
This solution has the same issues as Universal Coverage. Even assuming that Single Payer fixed some *financial* issues, it wouldn't directly fix most *quality* issues.

However, this limitation might end up being less significant than it appears. In countries where the government pays for most of the costs of health care, it typically directs a greater portion of the available money to prevention and primary care. As a result, both costs and health improve. For example, according to one study, your chances of dying an early death that could have been prevented are about 75 percent greater in the U.S. than in France,[270] where the government pays for a much larger share of care.

Regulation

The premise:
Relationships are sometimes too cozy between doctors and hospitals, or between doctors/hospitals and manufacturers of drugs or surgical products. As a result, care choices sometimes are based more on profits than on the best interests of patients.[271] Rules that prohibit, regulate, or mandate reporting of those relationships—and how much doctors are paid as a result—are intended to counter this tendency.

The limitations:
Doctors are usually fairly quick to figure out new rules and adapt to preserve their income. Without addressing the underlying mindset—that health care isn't focused on the patient—this behavior is unlikely to change.

Cost Controls

The premise:
The government pays nearly half the costs of health care and should negotiate lower prices.

The limitations:
This approach has a track record of failure.[272] For example, Medicaid, the shared federal and state health care program for the poor, has long required that it be given the lowest price that suppliers charge any customer. One exception allowed college health clinics to purchase contraceptives at a fraction of their retail price. This exception was eliminated in 2007.

To avoid having to give college pricing to Medicaid, manufacturers doubled or quadrupled their prices to the student health clinics.[273] Medicaid's costs did not drop—but a lot of college students could no longer afford birth control.

Similarly, when Medicare, the federal health program for the elderly and disabled, cuts the rates it pays, doctors avoid losing income by ordering more procedures. The government doesn't end up spending less in total, even though it pays less for each procedure.[274]

Given how often side effects and complications occur, the extra treatments probably have the unintended consequence of making many people's health worse.

Health Information Technology

The premise:
Lives and money can be saved by using EMRs (Electronic Medical Records), CPOE (Computerized Physician Order Entry—doctors' orders that are electronic rather than handwritten), artificial intelligence, and other computerized aids to help make decisions, manage and coordinate care, and keep records.

A patient's entire health history could be available anytime, anywhere. Smart computer systems could help to diagnose patients accurately and to identify treatment options that took individuals' unique characteristics into account. HIT (Health Information Technology) would bring record-keeping of your health information up to the level that your supermarket has been using for decades to track how many cans of soup it sells.

The limitations:
Many doctors prefer that people not see their own medical records.[275] Records people can't see won't help them better manage their care.

Additionally, unless health care changes its focus to be *to enable people to lead the lives they want,* all those electronic records could simply end up documenting a high volume of treatments that don't improve people's lives.

Comparative Effectiveness

The premise:
An impartial group evaluates treatments to figure out which ones work best. Individuals and their doctors select treatments that are likely to get good results. A focus on comparative effectiveness is long overdue and is a great step forward.

The limitations:
Doctors tend to ignore the results of such studies. For example, a big study in 2002 concluded that older drugs to treat high blood pressure worked better than new drugs that cost twenty times as much. However, six years later, doctors' prescribing practices had barely budged.[276]

Patients behave in a similar way: "Whether it's invasive back surgery, medical scans or expensive drugs, patients and doctors alike often refuse to believe that costly treatments aren't worth it."[277]

Most comparative effectiveness research focuses on clinical outcomes such as lowering blood pressure and doesn't answer questions about the impact of a treatment on people's ability to do the things they care about.

Further, because misdiagnoses are common, great comparative effectiveness research could result in your getting an excellent treatment for a disease you don't have.

Transparency

The premise:
"If you build it, they will come." That is, if information about quality and cost of care is broadly available, people will use it to make better decisions.

The limitations:
Individuals are at a huge power disadvantage, have limited knowledge about how health care works, may be kept in the dark about their own health, and so forth. For these reasons, they frequently don't have any meaningful way to use cost and quality information. In fact, research shows that people typically *don't* use this data when it is available.[278]

Information about costs would not have helped any of the people profiled to get better quality care. Information about quality might have helped if it directed people to other care providers or hospitals. However, quality measurements are typically focused on the delivery of acute interventions and typically don't consider issues such as misdiagnosis or the long-term consequences of hospital-related delirium.

Consumer-Directed Health Plans

The premise:
High-deductible health insurance plans will encourage consumers to be better health care shoppers, since they have to pay more of their own money before insurance kicks in.

The limitations:
Language has been hijacked here. Making people pay more money does not make something "consumer-directed."

A bigger issue is that the math simply doesn't support this idea. Just 5 percent of the people use 50 percent of the dollars spent on health care. And 20 percent use 81 percent of the health care dollars.[279] People whose care costs the most will probably exceed their high deductible in half a day's hospital stay, eliminating any incentive that having their own money at risk is supposed to create.

This plan shares the objections discussed under Transparency. It is unrealistic to think that people can make fact-based choices about doctors, hospitals, tests, and treatments when they are kept so thoroughly uninformed about their own health and health care.

It's not possible to empower people by saying, "You're empowered," when the health care system makes it clear in a hundred ways that they are not.

As one surgeon said, "Who comes up with this stuff? Any plan that relies on the sheep to negotiate with the wolves is doomed to failure."[280]

Pay for Performance

The premise:
Today, doctors get paid regardless of results. This approach is not effective. Paying doctors and hospitals for following best practices or for specific results will lead them to do the right thing. For example, hospitals and surgeons are measured on whether people get antibiotics in the 60 minutes before surgery, to prevent surgical infections. Doctors are measured on whether their patients with diabetes have had their blood sugar levels checked with the most useful test at least once in the past twelve months.

The limitations:
The measures that determine how much doctors get paid make little reference to the experience of the patient. Virtually all the measures evaluate one of three elements historically considered to define quality in health care:

- Structure, such as whether doctors send prescriptions electronically.
- Process, such as the percentage of heart attack patients who are prescribed beta blockers.
- Outcomes, such as the percentage of patients who were readmitted to the hospital within thirty days due to complications of care.[281]

These measures focus on the physicians' delivery of treatments. Sometimes patients are surveyed. However, it is rare to find systems that track how often the doctor performs various patient-focused tasks:

- Explains the pros and cons of different treatments, using consumer-friendly decision aids such as charts comparing the options.
- Helps people choose treatments that are the best fit with their values and preferences.
- Gives individuals their test results the day they are first available.
- Confirms that people can repeat the names of drugs prescribed, the reasons for taking them, and the dosing.
- Reviews patients' experience with drugs prescribed for chronic conditions, to ensure that the drugs are doing more good than harm.

As a result of the types of activities that are rewarded, Pay for Performance may not support the goal of making health care truly individual-centric.[282]

Focused Care

The premise:
Focused factories, an idea discussed by Regina Herzlinger of Harvard, applies an effective manufacturing concept to health care delivery.

The idea is that it is hopelessly inefficient for individual doctors and hospitals to try to address the full range of health care issues. Focusing instead on being spectacularly good at one thing—hernia repair or cataract surgery, for example—can yield huge quality and cost improvements.[283]

Michael Porter, also of Harvard, and Elizabeth Teisberg, at the University of Virginia, suggest a concept that seems related. They propose that doctors organize into groups that focus on one disease and compete with other groups on the results they deliver.

For instance, they might compete on lowering the percentage of people with asthma who end up in the emergency room or on reducing the percentage of people with diabetes who have to have a limb amputated.[284] The integration of care and the focus on results in terms that mean something to the people being treated are welcome features.

The limitations:
The focus is still largely on improving the delivery of treatments, rather than on enabling people to lead the lives they want. One significant issue is that many people have multiple medical conditions and can't be neatly divided up into disease buckets.[285]

Additionally, many issues cut across diseases and treatments, such as hospital-induced delirium and the difficulty people have getting their own medical information.

Accountable Care Organizations

The premise:
Selected doctors and hospitals work together to improve quality and cost of care for a specific group of patients. They get paid for getting better results at a lower cost.

The idea is to get the benefits of integrated, coordinated care providers such as the Mayo Clinic (where the doctors are all on salary and patients' electronic medical records are instantly available to all the doctors) when the players don't belong to one legal entity.

The limitations:
Issues are similar to those for Pay for Performance: how is quality of care defined? Are patients central or does the framework reflect traditional measures of structure, process, and outcomes?

Medical Homes

The premise:
A primary care doctor coordinates all care, using a team of nurses, administrative staff, and others. While primary care doctors have always had this role in theory, in practice they did very little coordination of care with specialists, management of overall wellness, and so forth.

Medical homes offer advantages not always found in other care models:

- They define clear processes for everything from scheduling appointments to reporting test results.
- They use Electronic Medical Records (EMRs).
- They coordinate with specialists, hospitals, and other providers.
- They coach people to better manage their own health.
- They track activities to ensure that preventive care is given, chronic conditions are managed, and the team does what it says it will do.[286]

Doctors' offices that follow the guidelines for medical homes will give people much more information and help than is typical today, and will treat them with more consideration. These are big wins.

The limitations:
Putting one doctor in charge doesn't shift the focus from doctors to you. Guidelines for medical homes do not cover topics such as improving the speed and accuracy of diagnosis and evaluating the results of treatments ordered to ensure that side effects are not swamping benefits.

In the end, the ultimate medical home shouldn't be your primary care doctor's office. It should be you, wherever you are—twenty-four hours a day, seven days a week. To get the best outcomes, care should center on you.

A study published in the *Annals of Family Medicine* discovered that medical homes delivered small improvements in several areas, but stayed the same or got worse in everything that patients evaluated, such as prompt access to care, coordination of care, and getting comprehensive care.[287]

Twelve fixes with the wrong starting point

As a doctor who writes a column in the *New York Times* commented in an article reporting on disappointing results from medical homes, "In working so hard to adopt changes on their patients' behalf, clinicians had temporarily lost their focus on the patients themselves."[288]

And that, in fact, is precisely the problem with all twelve improvement ideas listed here. There is very little evidence that they start from the basic premise that health care should meet patients' needs—that it should *enable people to lead the lives they want*. Very few of the twelve fixes would have made much of a difference for any of the people whose stories are told in this book.

Appendix B

An aside on the role of the patient

When Health Care Hurts describes danger spots to watch for and offers questions to ask and action steps to take to help you avoid being blindsided by unexpected problems as you seek the best that health care has to offer.

Patients have other roles, of course, and this note offers a brief nod in the direction of one of them: making choices that might reduce the number of occasions people have to interact with the health care system in the first place.

What else can patients do?

While it's true that health care professionals often accidentally cause harm, most of us aren't perfect at taking the steps needed to improve our health, either. Comic strips, always a great reflection of the culture, offer insight. Here is the dialog from a *Hagar the Horrible* comic:

Hagar: "My doctor said I have to make big changes in my diet . . . He said I have to switch from beer to water . . . and switch from fatty foods to fresh vegetables!"
Lucky Eddie: "Wow! What are you going to do?"
Hagar: "I'm going to switch doctors."[289]

Following in Hagar's footsteps, it turns out that fewer than 10 percent of us actually follow these basic recommendations:

- Eat 5 servings of fruit and vegetables daily.
- Exercise for 30 minutes 4-5 times a week.
- Drink moderately.
- Don't smoke.[290]

One writer noted, "Americans eat worse, exercise less and count on pills and doctors to bail them out more than the residents of any other country."[291]

Even hospital-acquired infections, adverse drug events, and other harm associated with health care delivery can sometimes be traced back to us.

Consider hospital-acquired infections. People pick up infections in hospitals less than once in six thousand encounters, and infections that cause deaths arise from less than one out of every fifty-nine thousand encounters.[292] That's no excuse for the infections, and it's no comfort at all to anyone who's been seriously injured or watched a family member die from one of these infections.

But most of the rest of us aren't perfect about not spreading germs, either. One research study found that 15 percent of us don't even wash our hands after using the toilet.[293]

You may spread infections yourself if you visit someone in the hospital. You put your unwashed hand on the doorknob, then on the soda or coffee machine, the elevator buttons, and the counters. If doctors and nurses come along next, they'll pick up whatever bugs you left, and they'll very efficiently pass them along to the next patient they see if they don't wash their hands.

If you're carrying nasty germs—or pick some up on your way to the patient room you're visiting—and then touch the patient, the guard rails on the bed, the blanket, the doorknob to the bathroom, the faucets on the sink, or anything else in the room, you could easily be the direct source of an infection that the patient picks up.

On a similar note, responsibility for some adverse drug events can be traced to patients who don't follow dosing instructions. For example, they may double up on doses and end up overdosing themselves. They may "borrow" drugs from other people—drugs that are inappropriate for them.

They may start or stop taking medicines abruptly when the drug dose needs to be ramped up or tapered off slowly. They may decide on their own to take a mix of current prescription drugs, old prescriptions drugs left over from a previous illness, and over-the-counter drugs—creating a stew of conflicting or excessive chemicals in their bloodstreams.

In other words, the responsibility for some of the illnesses and deaths that result from care delivery can be laid directly at the feet of patients and their families. Individuals are part of the health care delivery system even if this fact is not generally acknowledged. It might be helpful to rethink our expectation that doctors should be much more consistent and deliberate guardians of our health than we are.

Consider an analogy. In the fairy tale *The Fisherman and His Wife*, the fisherman's wife demands that he petition a magic fish (who is really an enchanted prince) for ever grander homes and loftier positions—king, emperor, and Lord. Each wish is granted, until the final one: she has gone too far, and the fisherman returns home to find her in the hovel in which they started.

We petition the enchanted princes—the doctors—to save us. But we may have gone too far, consuming a staggering amount of resources:

- One out of ten employed civilians works in health care.[294]
- Health care spending averages $8,915 per person per year.[295]
- More than 17 cents of each dollar in the economy goes to health care.[296]

Most experts think that the country can't afford this level of spending. Every dollar spent on health care means one less dollar for schools, roads, housing, and so forth. We have developed unrealistic expectations that doctors and the U.S. economy can't possibly meet. We may have accidentally replaced a desire for good health with a desire for acute interventions (medical treatments).

Business leader Paul Otellini noted: "From the 19th-century birth of clinics, medical technologies and specialty care, we have inherited two fundamental assumptions that no longer serve us well in the 21st century: 1) We wait for an illness or injury; 2) then we travel to a medical institution for an expert to repair things."

He continued, "We can no longer afford this pilgrimage to expensive and crowded medical centers for our every health care need. Nor can we relinquish all responsibility for our well-being to the doctors and caregivers who perform miracles every day to put us back together again."[297]

If we took better care of ourselves, perhaps half the volume of activity in the health care system would be eliminated because we simply wouldn't need treatment. That is, we would prevent most cases of diabetes, heart disease, and so forth.

This change would automatically reduce deaths caused by health care. For example, if people had only half as many hospital stays, there would be half as many opportunities for them to end up with hospital-related infections, blood clots, bedsores, delirium, and so forth.[298]

The lower volume of activity could also provide another benefit, giving the health care system more breathing space to use to fix the broken processes that harm so many Americans today.

Readers' Discussion Guide

Readers in discussion groups are welcome to select a subset of questions to answer; don't feel that you have to answer them all. Feel free to abstain from answering any questions that you are not comfortable addressing in a group. Also feel free to alter the personal details of any examples you give to protect the privacy of family and friends.

Chapter 1: "We have the best health care in the world"

1. Bob lived because his mother Shannon noticed obscure details—whether the drug in the syringe appeared clear or cloudy, for example—and spoke up. How does that event compare with your expectations about the role of patients (or their parents or other advocates) when they are hospitalized?

2. Christine died from an infection in an IV line. Her husband, Patrick, blames himself for not being more assertive and insisting that the hospital deal with the problem sooner. When a family member is in the hospital, who would you say ought to be responsible for the patient's well-being?

3. Louise's surgeon never considered the idea that her shoulder pain might be caused by a blood clot related to the surgery he performed. Have you had an experience in which you felt that a new problem

was a complication of treatment? How did you succeed in getting the doctor's attention to address the complication? Or, how would you proceed if you had such a problem in the future?

4. How does your experience support or contradict the picture painted about deaths and injuries caused by health care?

5. Do you think that medical errors, hospital-acquired infections, post-surgery blood clots, and adverse drug events are inevitable? (One might call this the "You can't make an omelet without breaking eggs" perspective.) Why or why not?

6. About 12 million people are harmed each year in America by the care they receive in the hospital. What do you feel an acceptable number is?

7. If you got into a conversation with someone who insisted that the U.S. has the best health care in the world, what would you say?

8. Only about half the leaders of hospital boards said that quality of care was one of their top two priorities. If you were on the board of a hospital, what top two priorities would you set for the hospital's CEO?

9. If you find yourself in the role of advocate for a family member who is hospitalized, which suggestions for being an advocate do you think you might act on? (Some of these are: find out what tests and treatments were ordered, write down questions in a notebook, ask questions when someone comes to do a test or give a treatment that wasn't ordered, track tests and treatments actually delivered, follow guidelines to help prevent infections and other complications of care, point out if the patient isn't eating or drinking, and call for help if the patient suddenly seems worse.) If you think there are some you wouldn't do, what arrangements might you make to get them taken care of?

10. If you knew that you were going to be hospitalized, who's the first person you would choose to act as your advocate? What characteristics do they have that make them a good choice?

Chapter 2: "You'll be fine once the doctor patches you up"

11. Mildred was hospitalized because she broke her hip. Her hip healed perfectly, but hospital-acquired delirium robbed her of much of her mental ability, and she ended up losing her apartment and living per-

manently in a skilled nursing unit as a result. Do you know people who developed delirium in the hospital? What impact do you think that experience had on their long-term well-being?

12. This chapter describes similarities between hospital ICUs and prison camps for terrorist suspects. How did you feel when you read that section? Why?

13. What might you do differently when a family member or friend is in the hospital, given what you've read about delirium?

14. Simple changes such as dimming the lights at night can help reduce delirium and its consequences. Have you experienced situations in which you concluded that simple, inexpensive changes on the part of care providers could make a huge difference in the patient's comfort or health? What would need to happen for these changes to be made?

15. Robert was prescribed a blood thinner after he had a stroke. All his doctors knew about this prescription, but they never discussed his risk of going blind as a result, even though his other medical conditions increased the odds of this complication. Have you had an experience where lack of coordination among doctors put your health at risk? What would you do differently next time to prevent serious problems?

16. Robert was almost completely deaf before he was given the blood thinner that caused him to go blind. For this reason, his loss of sight was an even greater tragedy than the loss of one sense normally is. If you have a disability now, how will you change how you talk with doctors to ensure that they fully consider the implications of any new treatments on your ability to function?

17. About a third of Medicare patients (people age 65-plus or disabled) end up back in the hospital within 90 days of being discharged. This chapter suggests dozens of things that can go wrong when patients come home from the hospital. (Some of these involve: drug errors, missing equipment or supplies, absent helpers, malnutrition or dehydration, not knowing what problems need immediate attention and how to get it, not knowing what activities are safe to do, and not following up with the doctor.) Have you experienced any gaps like these? What happened? If you could pay attention to only three issues when someone comes home from the hospital, which ones would you focus on?

18. The health care system tends to believe that people will be fine once the doctor addresses their immediate crisis—swaps out a broken hip for a new one, for instance. What would you say to someone who offers this perspective?

19. Doctors often view complications as inevitable. However, the vast majority are due to lapses such as failing to wash hands or failing to evaluate someone for risk of blood clots. How would you like your doctors to behave regarding complications of medical care?

Chapter 3: "Side effects are no big deal"

20. Alesandra obediently took all the drugs prescribed for her. Would you do the same thing in her shoes? Why or why not? If not, how would you go about safely changing your prescription regimen?

21. Lawrence nearly died of liver failure, a side effect of a medicine he was taking that did not become apparent for many years. A specialist had suggested three years earlier that his symptoms might be a drug side effect, but his doctor hadn't done anything to check out that possibility. How could you avoid finding yourself in a situation similar to Lawrence's—finding out years later that information known earlier could have saved you a lot of harm?

22. One patient out of four develops side effects within three months of starting a drug that they are expected to take for a long time. Have you had a treatment that caused side effects or complications that outweighed the benefits of the treatment? How quickly did the problem become evident? Who noticed the problem—the patient or the doctor? What could you do differently in similar situations in the future to get a better outcome faster?

23. The FDA often doesn't know as much about side effects as you might expect, for several reasons, including: the short time that drugs are tested, the small number of people on whom the drugs are tested, the tendency of doctors running the tests to downplay patients' reports of side effects, and the tendency of doctors to dismiss patients' complaints of side effects once the drug is on the market. Knowing that the FDA's data is limited, what will you do differently in the future when you think that you may be experiencing a drug side effect?

24. If you experienced a serious side effect, which of these would you notify: your doctor, the drug's manufacturer, and/or the FDA? Why?

25. The health care system often behaves as if *treating* a side effect or complication is as good as *preventing* it. What do you think?
26. What would you do if you were prescribed a drug that caused significant weight gain?

Chapter 4: "Treatments work for everyone"

27. Rebecca got worse as her doctor tried various medicines to treat her depression. Were you surprised to read that most drugs work in less than half the people who take them? How will this information change what you say or do when your doctor proposes giving you a prescription?
28. A four-box chart shows that any person getting any treatment will get one of four results. What can you do to help ensure that you land in the preferred box, where the treatment helps with the original problems and doesn't create any serious new ones?
29. In many cases, people are given treatments that are not a good match for them. For example, hip replacements suited for tall, middle-aged men were given mostly to women and the elderly, often causing serious problems. In another case, pacemakers addressed a problem that 40 percent of the people who got them didn't have. What might you do to ensure that the treatments you get are a good fit for you?
30. What would you do if your doctor prescribed a treatment without saying what it was for?
31. Do you feel that your job as the patient is to follow doctors' orders? Why or why not?

Chapter 5: "If you don't get better, it must be your fault"

32. Hannah was fed corn-based formulas that she could not tolerate. She nearly died as a result. Her doctors refused to consider the possibility that the formula was the problem and refused to authorize banked human milk for her. If you were in her mother's shoes, what would you have done at that point?
33. If no matter what you did in dealing with the health care system you were made to feel that you were wrong, what would you do?
34. The author compares the position that patients are in when they deal with the health care system to the position that American Indians

were in when they dealt with Europeans. What analogy captures how you feel when you deal with the health care system?

Chapter 6: "Doctors focus on the important stuff"

35. Don needed treatment for leukemia to save his life, but the treatment made him so weak that he nearly died, and then his hospitalization for that problem led to severe bedsores. Have you had an experience in which problems with health care just seemed to stack on top of each other, creating a downward spiral that was difficult or impossible to get out of? What would you do differently in dealing with a similar situation the next time?

36. Elaine noted that neither she nor Don realized that he had four serious bedsores, open down to the bone, until she caught a glimpse of one of them through a curtain as he was being treated. If you were in Elaine's shoes, when would you have expected the doctor or nurse to let you and your husband know about this complication?

37. Were you surprised to learn that Don still suffers from the effects of his bedsores ten years later? How will the knowledge that side effects and complications can have long-lasting impacts change what you say or do the next time you or a family member is in the hospital?

38. The author reported that the biggest problem she had after a bicycle accident was that gauze pads stuck to a large open wound, and all the healing tissue was torn off every time the bandages were changed. Do you think that it is the job of doctors or nurses to explain details about home care to patients, like the fact that non-stick bandages are available from specialty medical supply houses? Why or why not?

39. Doctors have spent years—sometimes decades—learning to be doctors. It's understandable that they may believe that the most important medical actions are the ones they take. Do you agree? Why or why not?

Chapter 7: "The diagnosis you get is correct"

40. The author describes having a brain fluid leak that was misdiagnosed as a middle ear infection. Have you had a medical problem that didn't seem to fit the doctor's expectations? What happened? What would you do if you faced such a situation in the future?

41. Although it is doctors who went to medical school, the author suggests that patients should be viewed as experts about their own symptoms and responses to treatments. What do you think?

42. Stacy was told that her overactive bladder problem was all in her head. It turned out that it was due to drinking way too much diet cola. Have you ever been diagnosed as having a psychological problem that later turned out to be a physical problem? How long did it take to correct the error? What might you do in the future if faced with a similar situation?

43. Amber was misdiagnosed in the emergency room as having diabetes when in fact she had a brain infection. What will you do if you are unsure whether the diagnostic test you've gotten accurately reflects your physical condition?

44. Have you had a diagnostic test that led the doctor down a path that turned out to be irrelevant? How was the mistake discovered? What were the consequences of that error?

45. Were you surprised to find out that tests often result in false positives, saying that someone has a disease when she doesn't? How will this information change what you do if your doctor tells you that a test shows that you have a serious medical condition?

Chapter 8: "You don't need to know what's going on."

46. A nurse in the emergency room told Michelle to sign her right leg with a marker, without telling her that the surgeon would operate on the leg with her signature on it. The leg that needed surgery was her left leg. If Michelle hadn't asked a question, she could have ended up with a big problem. Have you had a health care worker rush you through steps such as signing informed consent forms—or imply in some other way that you didn't really need to know what was happening? How did you respond? How would you respond in a similar situation in the future?

47. A health care expert said, "Health care systems have always transferred uncertainty and risk to the patient." What did he mean? In what ways is that view consistent or inconsistent with your experience of health care?

48. Tom was taken from his hospital room to the radiology department for a medical test he didn't know anything about. He insisted on

knowing what the test was, what its purpose was, and who ordered it. What would you do in a similar situation?

49. Jack spent so much time focused on his surgery for colon cancer that it never occurred to him to ask what recovery would be like. What would you most want to know concerning recovery if you had major surgery?

50. Charles didn't remember what the doctor said during an office visit. What two approaches are you most likely to try to help you remember what your doctor says? (Examples include: bring a list of questions, ask someone to come with you to take notes, take a pad of paper and pen so you can take notes, ask to be allowed to dress before receiving instructions, and record the visit on your smartphone.)

Chapter 9: "Medical records are for doctors"

51. Shannon's blood count had dropped so low that it could have been life-threatening. However, she didn't know it for another six weeks, because no one told her the results of her blood test. Have you had a medical condition worsen because you didn't know what your test results said? How might you avoid a similar situation in the future?

52. Do you make a point of finding out if your test results are normal or not? How easy is it for you to find out? How long does it typically take to get the results? How long do you think it should take?

53. Not hearing back about test results promptly can create stress for patients. What would you do in such a situation?

54. Janice's records in her doctor's office said that she wanted to have a laparoscopic cholecystectomy in her home. That's an operation to remove a gallbladder. She had talked with the doctor about having a lap pool in her home. Do you think that there might be errors in your medical records? What leads you to your conclusion?

55. How do you feel about having access to all your own medical records? Under what circumstances would you be interested in actually reading them? Have you ever needed old medical records and been unable to get them? What might you do differently the next time you need your records?

56. If you were going to get your medical records for just one event or condition, which one would it be? Why?

57. How might having a copy of your medical records help you?

Chapter 10: "Doctor knows best"

58. Terry was very clear with her surgeon that she did not want any anesthesia or mind-altering drugs during the operation to fix her broken wrist, because she had a paradoxical reaction to such drugs that led to extreme agitation and violence. The doctor ignored her comments and the nurse anesthetist said, "I think I know what's best for you; you're just a truck driver." Have you ever felt that your voice simply wasn't being heard when you were talking with medical professionals? What happened? What might you do differently in the future if confronted with a similar situation?

59. Five years later, Terry has only recovered about 30 percent of the use of her arm. One surgeon who reviewed her pre-surgical x-rays long after she was treated told her that she would almost certainly have healed perfectly well without any surgery. Have you concluded after the fact that a less aggressive or invasive treatment probably would have gotten you better results? How can you avoid getting into a situation where you find out too late that a less aggressive or less invasive treatment probably would have been better for you?

60. Because Terry is scared that doctors in the future might ignore her medical history and once again give her drugs that "hijack" her mind, she avoids all medical care and screening tests. If you found yourself in a situation similar to Terry's, would you make the same decision? Why or why not?

61. Carla was so sick that she wanted to die. Her pharmacist prepared a carefully researched report showing that almost all of her symptoms were probably due to side effects and drug interactions among the 13 prescriptions her doctor had put her on. Her doctor threw the report across the room at her and exclaimed, "I can't believe you'd insult me like this!" What would you do if you found yourself in this situation?

62. For patients to be meaningfully involved in their own care, researchers concluded that seven elements must be present. The first five reflect things they need to know: that they have a right to have a say, the medical issue in question, treatment options, pros and cons of each, and the odds of success of each. Sixth, the doctor needs to confirm that the patient does understand those five items. And seventh, the patient is asked what treatment he or she prefers. When you have talked with your doctor about a serious medical situation, are you

satisfied with how many of these elements were present? If not, what will you do differently in the future?

63. Have you ever decided to do something different from the doctor's initial suggestion? What led to your decision? How did the situation work out? If you have not had this experience, how would you go about getting a voice in the next decision you face about a major test or treatment?

64. One doctor writing in a medical journal said that neither the doctor nor the patient is the central figure; instead, they should both be viewed as stars revolving around a "common center of gravity." Do you agree? Why or why not? If you agree, what is that common center of gravity—the powerful force exerting a pull on both?

65. A third-grade teacher taught children about discrimination by treating half the students as if they could do no wrong and half as if they could do no right. (She switched their roles the next day.) Interestingly, the children did poorly on their schoolwork on the day they were treated as inferior and spectacularly well on the day they were treated as brilliant. Have you had an experience in which being treated dismissively by your doctor left you feeling less capable of managing your care? What might you do differently in the future to regain a sense of control and power about your health and health care?

66. Benjamin almost died of heart failure because his doctor first dismissed his symptoms and then took days to do tests and send him to a heart specialist. What would you do if you felt that you had a serious problem, but your doctor said you didn't?

67. Benjamin told his wife Theresa that he was doing what the doctor said, because that's what good patients do. What is your definition of a "good patient"?

68. Many research studies conclude that patients are reluctant to challenge their doctors. What could you do to help you feel more comfortable in talking with your doctor, if you believe that you need to question the plan your doctor has for you, or if you disagree with that plan and want to take a different approach to treatment?

69. Jonathan did not have surgery until eleven days after a spinal injury left him shrieking in pain. His doctor said that he would risk bleeding out if he had surgery any sooner, because Jonathan had recently taken a baby aspirin. However, the surgeon's delay left Jonathan at risk for paralysis, respiratory arrest, and neurological damage. Do

you believe that it is up to the doctor to decide what risks the patient will take? If not, what would you say to the surgeon if you were in a similar situation?

70. One study comparing two groups of people who were equally ill found that the group that got more treatment (surgery, for instance) ended up in worse health. How will this information change your approach to getting medical care?

71. Doctors often complain that insurance companies try to *limit* tests and treatments to foster their own financial interests rather than the patient's well-being. This chapter indicates that doctors may *order* tests and treatments to foster their own financial interests rather than the patient's well-being. With the insurance company saying one thing and the doctor saying another, how might you go about figuring out if a proposed test or treatment is in fact in your best interests or not?

72. Respected experts have concluded that about a third of the money spent on health care tests and treatments doesn't provide any benefit. In fact, the Mayo Clinic concluded that "a high percentage" of all tests and treatments may eventually be found not to help more than they hurt. How will this perspective change how you make decisions about what tests and treatments to get?

73. The author was admitted to the hospital as a teenager, with a severe breathing problem that left her unable to talk. What assumption do you think her mother was making when she decided to leave her child alone in the hospital and go back to work? What assumptions would you make in a similar situation?

74. Have you had an experience in which a doctor or nurse seemed more intent on maintaining authority than on meeting your needs? What happened? What would you do differently in the future if you faced a similar situation?

Chapter 11: How did we get here?

75. The author talks about three eras of health care. In the first one, public health agencies worked to clean up the water supply; in the second, doctors like TV's fictional Marcus Welby, MD took care of everything, saving lives by treating infectious diseases and other sudden-onset problems; in the third, individuals have to take charge

of their health to prevent and manage chronic conditions. How does this picture change how you think about your role vs. your doctors' roles in managing your health?

76. The author suggests that problems in health care arise from ten dangerous assumptions that might have made sense in earlier eras but cause a lot of harm today. Do you agree? Why or why not? (The ten assumptions are: we have the best health care in the world; you'll be fine once the doctor patches you up; side effects are no big deal; treatments work for everyone; if you don't get better, it must be your fault; doctors focus on the important stuff; the diagnosis you get is correct; you don't need to know what's going on; medical records are for doctors; and Doctor knows best.)

77. Identify one of the ten assumptions that has caused a problem for you. If you were in charge of health care for the United States, how would you address that assumption so that it wouldn't cause so much trouble for other people?

78. If the process for reporting test results is designed for doctors, people will hear about abnormal results when the doctor has a chance to talk with them, which can take days or weeks—or longer. If the process is designed for patients, people will get all their test results as soon as they are available. How do you think the reporting of test results should work? Why?

79. Even a simple process such as going to a doctor's appointment or getting a medical test has many steps, each of which presents opportunities to have something fall through the cracks. Can you think of a time where an unexpected problem arose with an office visit or test? What would you do differently in a similar situation in the future to try to prevent such a problem?

80. The author concludes that the purpose of the health care system today is *to deliver tests and treatments*. Based on your experience, what do you think the purpose of the health care system is today?

81. The author goes on to propose that the purpose of health care should be *to enable people to lead the lives they want*. What do you think it should be?

82. Dr. Don Berwick is quoted as saying, "I have come to believe that we—patients, families, clinicians, and the health care system as a whole—would be far better off if we professionals recalibrated our work such that we behaved with patients and families not as hosts in

the care system, but as guests in their lives." What does he mean by that? Do you agree with him?

Chapter 12: When health care is about you

83. Sarah developed a life-threatening infection shortly after she had surgery on her wrist. The doctors saved her life, although she lost the use of that arm and was unable to do many things that she cared about. In your opinion, did the doctors' job end with saving her life? Why or why not?

84. Have you had an experience in which you had trouble handling basic activities of daily living after getting medical treatment? What happened to make the situation improve?

85. Pick one change in research priorities that the author suggests will result from making health care focus more on meeting the individual's needs. (These are: improving diagnostic accuracy; assessing individuals' real-life risks; managing co-morbidities (multiple diseases in the same person); matching patients to treatments; communicating to reduce stress; eliciting behavior change; and finding the secrets of placebo responders.) Do you think that the change you picked is likely to help patients or not? What leads you to your conclusion?

86. What would you think about a health insurance plan that lets you select any treatment you want—as long as you first clearly understand the benefits and risks of three or four legitimate treatments for the condition? The information you would be given would include how success is defined for each treatment, how many people out of 100 get that successful result, whether the treatment will solve the problem forever, and so forth. Would you prefer a system like this or a system in which the doctor just makes the choice for you? What are the advantages and disadvantages of the approach you prefer?

87. What other changes do you think will take place if health care's purpose becomes *to enable people to lead the lives they want*, and you are treated with more respect?

Chapter 13: What will it take to fix health care?

88. What did you think when you saw the total number of deaths attributed to side effects and complications of health care?

89. The author compares the kind of attention that a handful or few hundred deaths from transportation or other accidents get to the lack of attention that hundreds of thousands or millions of deaths from health care get. Why do you think that there's such a difference? If you were in charge of health care for the U.S., how would you go about changing the fact that the harm health care causes seems to be accepted as a given?

90. The author says that it will take a revolution to fix the problems in health care. Why does she use the term "revolution"? Why does she compare efforts to change how patients are viewed to efforts that freed the slaves or granted women the right to vote?

91. The author attributes side effects and complications of care largely to choices that professionals in the health care system make. Do you agree? Why or why not?

92. Implicit in the book is the suggestion that the problem with health care isn't primarily financial; it's primarily about who has power— who gets to set the priorities and call the shots. Do you agree? Said another way, if there were suddenly enough money to pay for health care for everybody without any limitations, would that fix the problems identified in *When Health Care Hurts*?

93. Identify one way you will change how you deal with your health and health care, or how you will talk with others about health care, as a result of reading *When Health Care Hurts*.

Acknowledgments

People who read drafts of the manuscript and provided insightful feedback to help make this book more useful for you include: Amy Bewley, Jen Bewley, Maureen Boshier, Chuck Fager, Mary Ann Flatley, Cathryn Gunther, Alisa Isaac, Pat Iyer, Cathy Kushner, Joan MacLatchie, Jackie Murray, Bridget O'Brien, Bill Patrick, Bernie Steines, and Barbara Taptich.

Helene O'Brien deserves special mention and thanks: she provided thoughtful and comprehensive feedback on not one but two very different drafts of the complete manuscript.

The fact that the people named above were gracious enough to provide feedback does not mean that they agree with the views expressed. Any errors, of course, are mine.

I remain perpetually indebted to my husband, Stephen Brubaker, for his constant willingness to set aside his own pursuits with little notice and spend hours or days addressing the conceptual, technical, or design issue of the moment. Stephen designed the cover and the layout of *When Health Care Hurts*, took the photograph that appears on the back cover, designs my websites, and routinely serves as an excellent sounding board.

Notes

Chapter 1: "We have the best health care in the world"

1. Daniel R. Levinson, "Adverse Events in Hospitals: National Incidence Among Medicare Beneficiaries," Office of Inspector General, U.S. Department of Health & Human Services, November 2010.

See also Daniel R. Levinson, "Op-Ed Column: Medical Mistakes Plague Medicare Patients," Office of Inspector General, U.S. Department of Health & Human Services, 16 November 2010.

See also Stuart Wright, "Few Adverse Events in Hospitals Were Reported to State Adverse Event Reporting Systems," Office of Inspector General, U.S. Department of Health & Human Services, 19 July 2012.

2. Donald M. Berwick, plenary presentation titled "Mont Sainte-Victoire" at the Institute for Healthcare Improvement 18th Annual National Forum on Quality Improvement in Health Care, Orlando, FL, 12 December 2006. An IHI study found adverse events occurred in more than 35 percent of hospital stays. Since more than 37 million people are hospitalized each year, more than 12 million people are harmed.

See also David C. Classen, Roger Resar, Frances Griffin, Frank Federico, Terri Frankel, Nancy Kimmel, John C. Whittington, Allan Frankel, Andrew Seger, and Brent C. James, "'Global Trigger Tool' Shows That Adverse Events in Hospitals May Be Ten Times Greater Than Previously Measured," *Health Affairs*, April 2011.

3. See, for example, http://georgewbush-whitehouse.archives.gov/infocus/medicare/health-care/ which talks about "the world's best health care system."

Similarly, President George W. Bush, "State of the Union," January 2006, "Americans enjoy the best health care facilities and medical professionals in the world."

The Speaker of the U.S. House of Representatives, John Boehner, referenced "the best health care system in the world," according to Gail Russell Chaddock, in a *Christian Science Monitor* article, "Health Care Reform: After Big GOP Gains, Will It Be Repealed?" 03 November 2010.

Other politicians go even further: "The best health care system the world has ever known," is how Senator Richard Shelby of Alabama described U.S. health care, according to *Politico Live*, 07 June 2009, http://www.politico.com/blogs/politicolive/0609/Shelby_Obama_will_destroy_best_health_care_system_the_world_has_ever_known.html.

A press release from the Harvard School of Public Health is titled, "Most Republicans Think the U.S. Health Care System is the Best in the World. Democrats Disagree," 20 March 2008. It reports that 68 percent of Republicans draw this conclusion, while 32 percent of Democrats agree.

4.   This list is drawn from a variety of sources.

See Linda T. Kohn, Janet M. Corrigan, and Molla S. Donaldson, eds., Institute of Medicine, *To Err is Human: Building a Safer Health System*, Washington: National Academies, 2000.

See also Kristin Reed and Rick May, "HealthGrades Patient Safety in American Hospitals Study 2011," March 2011.

See also David C. Classen, Roger Resar, Frances Griffin, Frank Federico, Terri Frankel, Nancy Kimmel, John C. Whittington, Allan Frankel, Andrew Seger, and Brent C. James, "'Global Trigger Tool' Shows That Adverse Events in Hospitals May Be Ten Times Greater Than Previously Measured, *Health Affairs*, April 2011.

5.   Anahad O'Connor, "When Surgeons Leave Objects Behind," *New York Times*, 24 September 2012.

See also Katharine Greider, "Hospitals May Be the Worst Place to Stay When You're Sick," *AARP Bulletin*, 01 March 2012.

6.   See Notes 4 and 5 above.

7.   Committee on Identifying and Preventing Medication Errors, Philip Aspden, Julie Wolcott, J. Lyle Bootman, and Linda R. Cronenwett, eds., Institute of Medicine, *Preventing Medication Errors*, Washington: National Academies, 2006. A summary appears at http://www.iom.edu/~/media/Files/Report%20Files/2006/Preventing-Medication-Errors-Quality-Chasm-Series/medicationerrorsnew.pdf.

8.   Jerald Winakur, "What Are We Going To Do With Dad?" *Health Affairs*, July/August 2005.

9.   Wikipedia, "Ignaz Semmelweis," accessed 29 March 2014. http://en.wikipedia.org/wiki/Ignaz_Semmelweis.

10.   Howard Gleckman with John Carey, "Medicine's Industrial Revolution," *Business Week*, 29 May 2006. "For 150 years we have known that doctors with unwashed hands pass infections from patient to patient. The Centers for Disease Control & Prevention figures that 80 percent of hospital-acquired infections are transmitted this way, costing billions of dollars annually to treat and killing thousands of people."

11.   Barbara Starfield, "Is US Health Really the Best in the World?" *JAMA*, 26 July 2000. The author explains her methodology for calculating deaths caused by health care and concludes, "In any case, 225,000 deaths per year constitutes the third leading cause of death in the United States, after deaths from heart disease and cancer. Even if these figures are overestimated, there is a wide margin between these numbers of deaths and the next leading cause of death (cerebrovascular disease)."

See also Timothy J. Mullaney, "Business, Heal Health Care," *Business Week*, 14 August 2006. "It's no secret how messy the U.S. health-care industry is. Americans spend 16 percent of gross domestic product on health care, but quality is poor. Medical mistakes are the nation's third-leading killer."

12.   Liz Szabo, "Patient, Protect Thyself," *USA Today*, 04 February 2007. "Only about 35 percent of hospital employees consistently wash their hands each time they prepare to touch a patient," quoting the head of the Joint Commission, which accredits hospitals.

13.   Christopher Lee, "Studies: Hospitals Could Do More to Avoid Infections—Poor Hygiene, Operating Room Traffic, Antibiotic Use Are Cited," *Washington Post*, 21 November 2006. "Infections acquired in hospitals, which take a heavy toll on patients, arise mainly from poor hygiene in hospital procedures, not from how sick patients were when they were admitted, according to three new studies." (Other researchers make similar points about medical errors and adverse drug events.)

See also the U.S. Department of Health & Human Services at http://www.health.gov/hai/prevent_hai.asp, which notes, "Our ultimate goal should be the elimination of" health care-associated infections, implying that they are viewed as 100 percent preventable.

See also Nicholas Bakalar, "Prevention: Cameras Can Help Ensure Hand Washing," *New York Times*, 06 February 2012. "One hospital improved hand-washing rates from 10 percent to 90 percent by installing cameras at all hand-washing stations."

See also Marty Makary, "How to Stop Hospitals From Killing Us," *Wall Street Journal*, 21 September 2012.

See also Kevin Sack, "Swabs in Hand, Hospital Cuts Deadly Infections," *New York Times*, 27 July 2007.

See also Robert Langreth, "Clean Hands," *Forbes.com*, 19 June 2006. "'Hand-washing can be the most powerful weapon on earth,' says New York University infection expert Philip M. Tierno, yet studies show doctors often forget to do it. . . . Strict infection-control measures and prudent antibiotic use have let hospitals in the Netherlands avoid the resistant staph strains that plague most U.S. hospitals. . . . Resistant staph infections dropped 90 percent at the University of Pittsburgh Medical Center after it began testing incoming ICU patients for exposure to resistant staph strains and isolating carriers. 'It saves money—and lives. There is no reason why this shouldn't be implemented in a universal way,' says Carlene Muto, head of infection control at the medical center."

14.   See, for example, Atul Gawande, *The Checklist Manifesto*, New York: Metropolitan Books, 2009.

15.   "Data and Statistics: HAI Prevalence Survey," Centers for Disease Control and Prevention, http://www.cdc.gov/HAI/surveillance/, quoting a *New England Journal of Medicine* study, "Multistate Point-Prevalence Survey of Health Care-Associated Infections," published 27 March 2014.

16.   While Dr. Pronovost routinely updates his checklist to improve clarity, the five items listed here are representative of various versions of his checklist.

See Laura Landro, "The Secret to Fighting Infections," *Wall Street Journal*, 27 March 2011.

See also "A checklist to prevent infection," a section in "Deadly infections: How good is your hospital at preventing them?" *Consumer Reports* online, June 2011. http://www.consumerreports.org/cro/2012/12/deadly-infections/index.htm.

17.   Ellen Nolte and C. Martin McKee, "Measuring the Health of Nations: Updating an Earlier Analysis," *Health Affairs*, January/February 2008.

See also Ellen Nolte and C. Martin McKee, "In Amenable Mortality—Deaths Avoidable Through Health Care—Progress in the US Lags That of Three European Countries," *Health Affairs*, August 2012. This article reports that other countries reduced amenable death rates more rapidly than the U.S. does.

See also Jordan Rau, "Needs Improvement: U.S. Health Care Not Getting Better, Report Finds," *Kaiser Health News* blog, 18 October 2011. It reports on a Commonwealth Fund study that gave the U.S. health care system a grade of 64 out of 100. The score dropped slightly over several years. "As observed in previous scorecards, the US is not achieving the health outcomes or quality that should be possible with the resources the nation invests."

On a related note, the World Health Organization ranked the U.S. health care system 37th in the world overall. See World Health Organization, "World Health Organization Assesses the World's Health Systems," 21 June 2000. An overview of the study can be found at http://www.who.int/whr/2000/media_centre/press_release/en/index.html. In the first appendix, the U.S. ranking can be seen. Some analysts object to the study's approach to ranking. Even if this study is discounted, others paint a similar picture.

18.   John A. Heit, "Venous Thromboembolism Prophylaxis for the Medical Patient," Mayo Clinic, Rochester, MN, 2006.

19.   John A. Heit, "The Epidemiology of Venous Thromboembolism," Mayo Clinic, Rochester, MN, 2006.

See also Laura Landro, "In the Hospital, Facing a Scourge of Killer Clots," *Wall Street Journal*, 01 April 2009.

See also www.PreventDVT.org or North American Thrombosis Forum at www.natfonline.org.

20.   "Fact sheets: CMS final rule to improve quality of care during hospital inpatient stays," 02 August 2013, found at http://www.cms.gov/newsroom/mediareleasedatabase/fact-sheets/2013-fact-sheets-items/2013-08-02-3.html.

21.   Dr. Caprini offers an extensive website at www.venousdisease.com.

See also www.PreventDVT.org or www.natfonline.org, which offers an online assessment tool.

A more extensive document for doctors can be found at http://www.plasticsurgery.org/Documents/medical-professionals/patient-safety-resources/Caprini%20RAM.pdf.

22.   This list is adapted from the Mayo Clinic, "Diseases and Conditions, Deep Vein Thrombosis, Symptoms," http://www.mayoclinic.org/diseases-conditions/deep-vein-thrombosis/basics/symptoms/con-20031922, accessed 23 May 2014.

23.   Dr. Caprini offers an extensive website at www.venousdisease.com.

See also www.PreventDVT.org or www.natfonline.org, which offers an online assessment tool.

A more extensive document for doctors can be found at http://www.plasticsurgery.org/Documents/medical-professionals/patient-safety-resources/Caprini%20RAM.pdf.

24.   John A. Heit, "Venous Thromboembolism Prophylaxis for the Medical Patient," Mayo Clinic, Rochester, MN, 2006.

Another part of the equation is found in John A. Heit, "The Epidemiology of Venous Thromboembolism," Mayo Clinic, Rochester, MN, 2006.

See also Laura Landro, "In the Hospital, Facing a Scourge of Killer Clots," *Wall Street Journal*, 01 April 2009.

See also www.PreventDVT.org or North American Thrombosis Forum at www.nat-fonline.org.

25.   Gina Maiocco, "DVT Prevention for the Obese Patient: Evidence-Based Nursing Interventions," *Bariatric Nursing and Surgical Patient Care*, 06 December 2008.

26.   Marshall Allen, "First Do No Harm," *Washington Monthly*, March/April 2011.

27.   Daniel R. Levinson, "Hospital Incident Reporting Systems Do Not Capture Most Patient Harm," U.S. Department of Health & Human Services, January 2012.

28.   "Rank Order—Life Expectancy at Birth," *CIA World Factbook*, 23 March 2014.

29.   Ashish K. Jha and Arnold M. Epstein, "Hospital Governance and the Quality of Care," *Health Affairs* online 06 November 2009.

30.   Robert Pear, "New System for Patients to Report Medical Mistakes," *New York Times*, 22 September 2012.

31.   The Institute for Healthcare Improvement (http://www.ihi.org/ihi/about), found-ed and formerly led by Dr. Don Berwick, is seen by many to be leading the charge. See his book *Escape Fire* (Jossey-Bass, 2003) for some of his extraordinarily moving speeches at IHI's annual convention focused on reducing the harm health care does to patients.

32.   Lucian Leape and Karen Davis, "To Err Is Human; To Fail to Improve Is Uncon-scionable," Commonwealth Fund, 16 August 2005.

33.   Kevin Sack, "Government Reports Criticize Health Care System," *New York Times*, 07 May 2009.

34.   David C. Classen, Roger Resar, Frances Griffin, Frank Federico, Terri Frankel, Nancy Kimmel, John C. Whittington, Allan Frankel, Andrew Seger, and Brent C. James, "'Global Trigger Tool' Shows That Adverse Events in Hospitals May Be Ten Times Greater Than Previously Measured," *Health Affairs*, April 2011.

35.   Tara F. Bishop, Andrew M. Ryan, and Lawrence P. Casalino, "Paid Malpractice Claims for Adverse Events in Inpatient and Outpatient Settings," *JAMA*, 15 June 2011. Roughly equal numbers of malpractice claims were paid for inpatients and for outpatients in the U.S. in the five years ending in 2009. The authors suggest that health care may result in as much harm outside of hospital settings as inside.

See also Tara Parker-Pope, "Testing Mistakes at the Family Doctor," *New York Times*, 14 August 2008. The article says that "medical errors or adverse events in family practices occur in about one in four patient visits," without identifying the relevant research.

36.   Daniel R. Levinson, "Hospital Incident Reporting Systems Do Not Capture Most Patient Harm," U.S. Department of Health & Human Services, January 2012.

See also Robert Pear, "Report Finds Most Errors at Hospitals Go Unreported," *New York Times*, 06 January 2012.

Chapter 2: "You'll be fine once the doctor patches you up"

37.   E. Wesley Ely, "ICU Delirium Epidemiology, Monitoring, & Management," slide presentation, 2006. http://www.mc.vanderbilt.edu/icudelirium/docs/ICU_slides_02_2006.pdf.

38.   This general response is confirmed by the following description in an article by

Laura Landro, "Hospitals Combat an Insidious Complication," *Wall Street Journal*, 17 October 2007: "When someone is in the hospital, it is common to get confused and delirious, but the tradition in medicine has been to say, 'Don't worry if Grandma or Grandpa is confused, it's no big deal'. But it is a major public-health problem that has to be addressed."

39.   From http://www.mc.vanderbilt.edu/icudelirium/overview.html, reporting on the work of the ICU Delirium and Cognitive Impairment Study Group, run by Dr. Wes Ely of Vanderbilt University Medical Center. This quotation (no longer online) appeared under "Prevalence and Clinical Relevance," downloaded 20 February 2011: "Critically ill patients are at great risk for the development of delirium in the ICU. With more than 8 out of 10 ventilated patients experiencing delirium, this is one of the most frequent forms of organ dysfunction experienced by critically ill patients. Despite this prevalence, delirium (usually in the hypoactive state) remains unrecognized in 66 percent to 84 percent of patients whether they be in the ICU, hospital ward, or emergency department."

40.   E. Wesley Ely, "ICU Delirium Epidemiology, Monitoring, & Management," slide presentation, 2006. http://www.mc.vanderbilt.edu/icudelirium/docs/ICU_ slides_02_2006.pdf. Dr. Ely notes that it usually takes far less than 30 seconds to diagnose delirium because it becomes evident with the answers to just a few questions.

41.   The author has spoken to audiences ranging from two people to fifteen hundred people. All audiences, when asked what location has the characteristics listed, rapidly came up with both correct answers.

Characteristics of prison camps for terrorist suspects were also identified by Chuck Fager, then Director, Quaker House, e-mail to the author, 12 June 2008.

See also Alfred McCoy, *A Question of Torture*, New York: Henry Holt, 2006. Prisoners held for interrogation may be subjected to either sensory deprivation or sensory overload. The effect is similar.

The fact that the characteristics listed are also representative of a hospital ICU was confirmed in dozens of conversations with hospital administrators, nurses, and doctors.

See also "Study: Lack of Sleep Hurts ICU Patients," *FierceHealthcare*, 18 December 2007, which summarizes a study that concluded in part, "Patient sleep is frequently disrupted by excessive light and noise, a lack of cues as to time of day . . . "

42.   Chuck Fager, then Director, Quaker House, e-mail to the author, 12 June 2008. Terrorist suspects may be drugged when in transit from one location to another, but are typically not drugged while being held for interrogation.

43.   Patient education brochure prepared by the ICU Delirium and Cognitive Impairment Study Group, run by Dr. Wes Ely of Vanderbilt University Medical Center, at http:// www.mc.vanderbilt.edu/icudelirium/docs/delirium_education_brochure.pdf, downloaded 29 March 2014.

44.   Judith Graham, "After Hospitalization, Mental Trouble for Elderly Patients," *New York Times*, 23 March 2012.

45.   Patient education brochure prepared by the ICU Delirium and Cognitive Impairment Study Group, run by Dr. Wes Ely of Vanderbilt University Medical Center, at http:// www.mc.vanderbilt.edu/icudelirium/docs/delirium_education_brochure.pdf, downloaded 29 March 2014.

46.   E. Wesley Ely, "ICU Delirium Epidemiology, Monitoring, & Management," slide presentation, 2006. http://www.mc.vanderbilt.edu/icudelirium/docs/ICU_ slides_02_2006.pdf.

47.   Laura Landro, "Hospitals Combat an Insidious Complication," *Wall Street Journal*, 17 October 2007, reporting on Dr. Ely's work. This article stops short of the supposition I have added, that patients interpret their circumstances to mean that they are being held prisoner. This is a theme in a number of accounts of people suffering PTSD (post-traumatic stress disorder) after bouts of delirium in hospitals. A former U.S. Air Force pilot, for example, told me that he had believed that he was being held captive by the Cubans, when he was seriously ill in the hospital. (He had been a fighter pilot decades earlier during the Cuban missile crisis.) His account is not unusual.

See also Gina Kolata, "A Tactic to Cut I.C.U. Trauma: Get Patients Up," *New York Times*, 12 January 2009. "Researchers say they are alarmed by what they are finding as they track patients for months or years after an I.C.U. stay. Patients, even young ones, can be weak for years. Some have difficulty thinking and concentrating or have post-traumatic stress disorder and terrible memories of nightmares they had while heavily sedated."

See also Pam Belluck, "Hallucinations in Hospital Pose Risk to the Elderly," *New York Times*, 20 June 2010.

48.   Laura Landro, "Hospitals Combat an Insidious Complication," *Wall Street Journal*, 17 October 2007.

49.   Laura Landro, "Hospitals Combat an Insidious Complication," *Wall Street Journal*, 17 October 2007.

This conclusion is based on anecdotal evidence at the moment. However, the anecdotal evidence is strong. "Preliminary evidence shows that each day spent in a delirious state increases the risk of long-term cognitive impairment by 35 percent. While many factors can contribute to such impairment, several studies have shown links between delirium, declining mental function and eventual dementia, says Dr. Ely. Patients can end up 'in their own little hell,' he says, where they have trouble thinking straight or doing simple tasks like balancing a checkbook. The causes of so-called acquired long-term cognitive impairment after ICU stays are being investigated in two large studies funded by Veterans Affairs and the National Institutes of Health."

The article tells of a busy mid-career professional whose IQ dropped from 145 before an ICU stay to 110 afterwards—a drop of nearly 25 percent. This 40-something woman was forced to retire from her job because she could no longer do it, "and an MRI scan showed atrophy in her brain similar to what might appear in an 80-year-old woman with dementia, the progressive and permanent loss of memory and cognition."

See also Sharon K. Inouye, "Delirium in Older Persons," *New England Journal of Medicine*, 16 March 2006.

See also Laura Landro, "Changing Intensive Care to Improve Life Afterward," *Wall Street Journal*, 15 February 2011. "Research conducted in recent years shows that 50 percent to 80 percent of people who leave the ICU later suffer from long-term cognitive impairment that appears to be related to how long they were delirious in the hospital, Vanderbilt says."

See also Gina Kolata, "A Tactic to Cut I.C.U. Trauma: Get Patients Up," *New York Times*, 12 January 2009. "Researchers say they are alarmed by what they are finding as they track patients for months or years after an I.C.U. stay. Patients, even young ones, can be weak for years. Some have difficulty thinking and concentrating or have post-traumatic stress disorder and terrible memories of nightmares they had while heavily sedated."

50.   Laura Landro, "Hospitals Combat an Insidious Complication," *Wall Street Jour-

nal, 17 October 2007. The article reports on two hospitals that put simple plans in place that "all but eliminated cases of delirium."

51.   Robert Preidt, "Using Earplugs Eases ICU Patients' Confusion: Study," *Health Day*, 07 May 2012. "Starting to use earplugs within the first 24 hours after admission to the ICU decreased patients' risk for delirium or confusion by more than 50 percent."

52.   "Health Policy Brief: Care Transitions," *Health Affairs*, 13 September 2012. "One of the biggest barriers to smoother care transitions is the fact that primary care physicians often have little or no information about their patients' hospitalizations. A review of the literature published in the *Journal of the American Medical Association* in 2007 found that physicians had received a hospital discharge summary about their patients, and had it on hand, in only 12-34 percent of first postdischarge visits. Even when discharge summaries are received, they often lack key information, such as test results, treatment course, discharge medications, and follow-up plans," making it very hard to follow up effectively.

See also Anthony Shih, Karen Davis, Stephen Schoenbaum, Anne Gauthier, Rachel Nuzum, and Douglas McCarthy, "Organizing the U.S. Health Care Delivery System for High Performance," ed. Martha Hostetter, The Commonwealth Fund, 7 August 2008. "Poor communication and lack of clear accountability for a patient among multiple providers lead to medical errors."

53.   In previous accounts, I have used the pseudonym "Joan" for this patient. However, in this chapter another story involving a different individual named Joan immediately precedes this one. To avoid confusing the reader, I have assigned a new pseudonym, "Linda," to the patient in the third story in this chapter.

54.   Stephen F. Jencks, Mark V. Williams, and Eric A. Coleman, "Rehospitalizations among Patients in the Medicare Fee for Service Program," *New England Journal of Medicine*, 02 April 2009.

55.   "Health Policy Brief: Care Transitions," *Health Affairs*, 13 September 2012.

Chapter 3: "Side effects are no big deal"

56.   Sandra G. Boodman, "Are Doctors To Blame?" *Washington Post*, 27 May 2008. This article reports on a Mayo Clinic study that showed that upon hospital discharge only 11 percent of patients said that they had been warned about side effects of new medicines prescribed for them. Many other studies show similar numbers.

57.   Tejal K. Gandhi, Saul N. Weingart, Joshua Borus, Andrew C. Seger, Josh Peterson, Elisabeth Burdick, Diane L. Seger, Kirstin Shu, Frank Federico, Lucian L. Leape, and David W. Bates, "Patient Safety: Adverse Drug Events in Ambulatory Care," *New England Journal of Medicine*, 17 April 2003.

See also Tejal K. Gandhi and Thomas H. Lee, "Patient Safety Beyond the Hospital," *New England Journal of Medicine*, 08 September 2010.

58.   Charlene Laino, "Is Your Medicine Cabinet Making You Fat?" http://www.web-md.com/a-to-z-guides/features/is-your-medicine-cabinet-making-you-fat, accessed 29 March 2014.

59.   Tejal K. Gandhi, Saul N. Weingart, Joshua Borus, Andrew C. Seger, Josh Peterson, Elisabeth Burdick, Diane L. Seger, Kirstin Shu, Frank Federico, Lucian L. Leape, and David

W. Bates, "Patient Safety: Adverse Drug Events in Ambulatory Care," *New England Journal of Medicine*, 17 April 2003.

See also Tejal K. Gandhi and Thomas H. Lee, "Patient Safety Beyond the Hospital," *New England Journal of Medicine*, 08 September 2010.

60.   Beatrice A. Golomb, John J. McGraw, Marcella A. Evans, and Joel E. Dimsdale, "Physician Response to Patient Reports of Adverse Drug Effects," *Drug Safety*, August 2007.

61.   Ibid.

62.   Ibid.

63.   Mary Duenwald, "Is Your Medicine Cabinet Making You Fat?" *New York Times*, 16 August 2005.

64.   Beatrice A. Golomb, John J. McGraw, Marcella A. Evans, and Joel E. Dimsdale, "Physician Response to Patient Reports of Adverse Drug Effects," *Drug Safety*, August 2007.

65.   See, for example, Siri Carpenter, "Is Your Parent Over-Medicated?" *Prevention*, December 2008.

66.   Duff Wilson, "Harvard Medical School in Ethics Quandary," *New York Times*, 04 March 2009.

67.   Gary Ahlquist, Charles Beever, Rick Edmunds, and David G. Knott, "Consumer and Physician Readiness for a Retail Healthcare Market: Changing the Basis of Competition," Booz Allen Hamilton Consumerism Survey Report, 2007.

68.   Gardiner Harris, "Prosecutors Plan Crackdown on Doctors Who Accept Kickbacks," *New York Times*, 04 March 2009.

See also Tracy Weber and Charles Ornstein, "What the Doctor Ordered: Patients Should Know If Their Doctors Get Paid by Drug Firms," *Los Angeles Times* online, 08 September 2011.

69.   Jerry Gurwitz, Mark Monane, Susan Monane, and Jerry Avorn, *Long-Term Care Quality Letter*, Brown University, 1995.

See also Melinda Beck, "Searching for Side Effects," *Wall Street Journal*, 31 January 2012.

See also Sharon Begley, "One Word Can Save Your Life: No!" *Daily Beast*, 14 August 2011. The subtitle reads, "New research shows how some common tests and procedures aren't just expensive, but can do more harm than good." Drugs are not the only treatments that have downsides. "A study on stents—devices designed to prop open blocked arteries in the brain, with the aim of preventing strokes— was abruptly halted when it was found that subjects who received the stents actually suffered twice as many strokes as the subjects in the control group."

70.   Beatrice A. Golomb, John J. McGraw, Marcella A. Evans, and Joel E. Dimsdale, "Physician Response to Patient Reports of Adverse Drug Effects," *Drug Safety*, August 2007.

71.   Ethan Basch, "The Missing Voice of Patients in Drug-Safety Reporting," *New England Journal of Medicine*, 11 March 2010.

72.   Ibid.

73.   Estimates of deaths due to side effects of medicines vary; two studies are highlighted below.

Saul Weingart, Ross McL. Wilson, Robert W. Gibberd, and Bernadette Harrison, "Epidemiology of Medical Error," *BMJ*, 18 March 2000. Adverse drug events among people not in hospitals caused 17 million emergency department visits.

Frank R. Ernst and Amy J. Grizzle, "Drug-Related Morbidity and Mortality: Updating the Cost-of-Illness Model," *Journal of the American Pharmaceutical Association*, March/April 2001: side effects of drugs each year led to 18,703,833 ER visits annually.

74.   Leila Abboud, "Largest Ever Studies On Drugs for Depression, Schizophrenia Could Transform Treatment," *Wall Street Journal*, 27 July 2005.

See also National Library of Medicine, AHRQ Comparative Effectiveness Reviews, "Off-Label Use of Atypical Antipsychotic Drugs: A Summary for Clinicians and Policy-makers," 12 July 2007, available at www.effectivehealthcare.ahrq.gov. About 3 out of every 10 people taking one psychiatric drug, Xyprexa, gained at least 7 percent of their baseline weight (14 pounds for someone who weighs 200 pounds). An update at http://www.effectivehealthcare.ahrq.gov/search-for-guides-reviews-and-reports/?pageaction=displayproduct&productID=1193 dated 01 August 2012 reports that weight gain is a side effect for 1 in 3 people taking Xyprexa.

75.   "Gaining Weight? It Could Be Your Medication," *Johns Hopkins Health Alerts*, http://www.johnshopkinshealthalerts.com/alerts/nutrition_weight_control/medication-weight-gain_5954-1.html www.johnshopkinshealthalerts.com (no longer online).

76.   Mary Duenwald, "Is Your Medicine Cabinet Making You Fat?" *New York Times*, 16 August 2005. Although two articles referenced in this chapter have the same headline, they are different articles.

77.   Kathleen Zelman, "Lose Weight, Gain Tons of Benefits," http://www.webmd.com/diet/features/lose-weight-gain-tons-of-benefits, accessed 29 March 2014.

78.   Ethan Basch, "The Missing Voice of Patients in Drug-Safety Reporting," *New England Journal of Medicine*, 11 March 2010.

79.   Mary Duenwald, "Is Your Medicine Cabinet Making You Fat?" *New York Times*, 16 August 2005.

80.   "Kaiser Health Tracking Poll," Kaiser Family Foundation, February 2009. When asked, "Do you currently take any prescription medicine on a daily basis, or not?" 49 percent said yes, 50 percent said no, and 1 percent declined to answer or did not know.

81.   Barry Meier, "Pain Pills Add Cost and Delays to Job Injuries," *New York Times*, 02 June 2012.

82.   Orly Avitzur, "Be Wary of Narcotics to Treat Back Pain," *Consumer Reports*, May 2009.

Chapter 4: "Treatments work for everyone"

83.   http://www.thennt.com/nnt/antibiotics-for-clinically-diagnosed-acute-sinus-itis/, accessed 29 March 2014.

Researchers use a statistic called Number Needed to Treat (NNT) to clarify how many people have to take a drug for one person to benefit. NNT is explained further on a website, www.nntonline.net, run by Dr. Chris Cates. Dr. Cates has created a computer program to help doctors understand how to translate research results into more meaningful information to help them better practice medicine.

84.   "Lyrica Significantly Reduced Pain and Helped Patients Manage the Symptoms of

Fibromyalgia, Data Show," Press release, Pfizer, 01 May 2007. "Significantly more patients treated with Lyrica reduced their pain by 50 percent or more compared with placebo. Of those patients taking 600mg of Lyrica a day, 30 percent said their pain was cut in half or better; 27 percent of those taking 450mg a day and 24 percent of those taking 300mg also reported this level of pain relief. Of those taking placebo, 15 percent reported pain reduction of 50 percent or greater."

See also Lee Bowman, "Study: Diabetes drug cuts risk of disease," Scrips Howard News Service, 18 September 2006, reporting on a study at McMaster University in Ontario, Canada involving 5,269 patients at 191 sites in 21 countries. Avandia "normalized glucose levels in 51 percent of those who took it, compared with 30 percent in the placebo group."

See also John Carey, "Do Cholesterol Drugs Do Any Good?" *Business Week*, 16 January 2008. "Difficult risk-benefit questions surround most drugs. . . . One dirty little secret of modern medicine is that many drugs work only in a minority of people."

85.   Andrew Pollock, "FDA Approves a Drug for Hot Flashes," *New York Times*, 28 June 2013. (Also published as "Rejecting Advisory Panel's Finding, F.D.A. Approves a Drug for Hot Flashes," *New York Times*, 29 June 2013.)

See also David H. Freedman, "The Triumph of New-Age Medicine," *Atlantic*, July 2011. This article notes that "most approved drugs do only a little better than a placebo. . . . A number of studies have indicated, for example, that most antidepressants don't do better than placebos, but patients filled more than 250 million prescriptions for them in 2010."

Different studies have come to different conclusions about antidepressants. Generally, when they include only people who are more severely depressed, they conclude that the drugs help as much as 75 percent of the time. But they are often prescribed for people who don't fit that profile.

See also Donald W. Light, *The Risks of Prescription Drugs*, New York: Columbia University, 2010. Professor Light is a researcher with impressive credentials, based at the University of Medicine & Dentistry of New Jersey. He has concluded that 85 percent of new prescription drugs don't offer any benefits to patients.

See also Brian Spear, "Clinical Application of Pharmacogenetics," *Trends in Molecular Medicine*, 30 April 2001. According to this researcher, drugs for specific conditions work the following percentages of the time:

Alzheimer's	30%
Asthma	60%
Cancer	25%
Cardiac arrhythmias	60%
Depression	62%
Diabetes	57%

Some of his numbers seem optimistic when compared to those found in other studies. And, as noted in the text, one has to know what it means to say that a particular drug "works"—it may mean that people get only a small improvement, not that the problem goes away.

86.   Roni Caryn Rabin and Nicholas Bakalar, "Hazards: A Pacemaker is Found to

Carry Risk," *New York Times*, 20 June 2011, reporting on a study in the *Archives of Internal Medicine*.

87. Jerome Groopman and Pamela Hartzband, "Designing a Smarter Patient," *Wall Street Journal*, 24 September 2011. This article explains that without treatment, about 3 out of 100 patients with high cholesterol will have a heart attack over the course of ten years; with treatment with a statin, 2 patients will have heart attacks. Using these numbers, 100 people would have to take the drug for 10 years to avoid one heart attack.

88. John Carey, "Do Cholesterol Drugs Do Any Good?" *Business Week*, 17 January 2008. Researchers use a statistic called Number Needed to Treat (NNT) to clarify how many people have to take a drug for one person to benefit. Often, "The NNTs are large. Take Avandia, GlaxoSmithKline's drug for preventing the deadly progression of diabetes. The blockbuster, with $2.6 billion in U.S. sales in 2006, made headlines in 2007 when an analysis of clinical trial data showed it increased the risk of heart attacks. The largely un-told story: There's little evidence the drug actually helps patients. Yes, Avandia is very good at lowering blood sugar, just as statins lower cholesterol levels. But that doesn't translate into preventing the dire consequences of diabetes, including heart disease, strokes, and kidney failure. Clinical trials 'failed to find a significant reduction in cardiovascular events even with excellent glucose control,' wrote Dr. Clifford J. Rosen, chair of the Food & Drug Administration committee that evaluated Avandia, in a recent commentary in the *New England Journal of Medicine*. 'Avandia is almost the poster child for everything wrong with our system,' says UCLA's Hoffman. 'Its NNT is close to infinite.'"

NNT is explained further on a website, www.nntonline.net, run by Dr. Chris Cates.

On a related note, see Tara Parker-Pope, "A Call for Caution in the Rush to Statins," *New York Times*, 18 November 2008. She summarizes a study: "Only 1.8 percent of the subjects who took a placebo had a major cardiovascular problem during the study period. Among statin users, 0.9 percent did. In other words, the absolute risk of a serious cardiovascular problem (as opposed to the relative risk) was reduced by less than one percentage point."

See also John Carey, "Smarter Patients, Cheaper Care?" *Business Week*, 22 June 2009. The article is subtitled, "Better-informed medical decisions could cut billions in health-care costs as patients opt for cheaper treatments." Once patients understand the small ben-efit that many treatments confer, they elect not to get them.

See also Laura Landro, "Weighty Choices, in Patients' Hands," *Wall Street Journal*, 04 August 2009: "Studies show that when patients understand their choices and share in the decision-making process with their doctors, they tend to choose less-invasive and less-expensive treatments than they would have otherwise received."

89. Jeanne Lenzer, "Most People Who Take Blood Pressure Medication Possibly Shouldn't," *Slate*, 14 August 2012. The article reports on a study by the Cochrane Collabo-ration, which is an independent organization.

90. Gina Kolata, "Drug That Stops Bleeding Shows Off-Label Dangers," *New York Times*, 18 April 2011.

91. John Carey with Amy Barrett, "Is Heart Surgery Worth It?" *Business Week*, 18 July 2005. As an example of complications, according to Dr. Nortin Hadler of the University of North Carolina, coronary bypass surgery carries a 1-2 percent risk of death during the surgery and up to a 40 percent chance of permanent mental decline.

92. Steve Connor, "Glaxo Chief: Our Drugs Do Not Work on Most Patients," *Inde-pendent* (UK), 08 December 2003.

93.   Photo credit for four licensed images of faces: ©Mary Jackson | Dreamstime.com, #10866569, licensed and downloaded 27 March 2014.

94.   Steve Connor, "Glaxo Chief: Our Drugs Do Not Work on Most Patients," *Independent* (UK), 08 December 2003.

See also notes earlier in this chapter which detail other researchers' agreement with this point. This fact is well known in industry circles; executives typically don't say so publicly.

95.   "Script Your Future" campaign, National Consumers League, scriptyourfuture.org, accessed 29 March 2014.

96.   "Taking Medicine Is an Important Part of Staying Healthy," *Aetna Member Essentials*, May 2009. This view is representative of the industry.

On a related note, entire businesses focus on helping pharmaceutical companies drive compliance. The website of one of these, Consumer Health Information Corporation, says at http://www.consumer-health.com/services/srv_pharm.php that they have "helped product managers reach goals they never thought possible. Our team of experts develop a patient adherence strategy for the product. The results have led to astounding success for product managers." It highlights this statement: "Our programs have increased a product's ROI (return on investment) up to 50 percent." Note that there is no suggestion that success might be measured in terms of improving patients' health.

97.   Barry Meier, "In Medicine, New Isn't Always Improved," *New York Times*, 25 June 2011.

98.   Sundeep Khosla, "Increasing Options for the Treatment of Osteoporosis," *New England Journal of Medicine*, 12 August 2009.

99.   "Your Health: How Do You Score on Taking Your Medicine?" *Kiplinger's Retirement Report*, August 2011.

See also Tara Parker-Pope, "Keeping Score on How You Take Your Medicine," *New York Times*, 21 June 2011.

100.   "Preference-Sensitive Care," Dartmouth Atlas Project Topic Brief, downloaded 17 October 2012, available at http://www.dartmouthatlas.org/downloads/reports/preference_sensitive.pdf.

101.   Barry Meier, "Metal Hips Failing Fast, Report Says," *New York Times*, 15 September 2011.

Chapter 5: "If you don't get better, it must be your fault"

102.   Lucian L. Leape, Miles F. Shore, Jules L. Dienstag, Robert J. Mayer, Susan Edgman-Levitan, Gregg S. Meyer, and Gerald B. Healy, "Perspective: A Culture of Respect, Part 1: The Nature and Causes of Disrespectful Behavior by Physicians, *Academic Medicine*, July 2012. Six of the seven authors are doctors at Harvard.

103.   Owen MacDonald, "Disruptive Physician Behavior," American College of Physician Executives via QuantiaMD, 15 May 2011.

104.   Ibid.

105.   Todd Ackerman, "Saving Babies' Lives, Ounce by Ounce," *Houston Chronicle*, 15 August 2011.

106.   Lucian L. Leape, Miles F. Shore, Jules L. Dienstag, Robert J. Mayer, Susan Edgman-Levitan, Gregg S. Meyer, and Gerald B. Healy, "Perspective: A Culture of Respect,

Part 1: The Nature and Causes of Disrespectful Behavior by Physicians, *Academic Medicine*, July 2012.

Chapter 6: "Doctors focus on the important stuff"

107. "HealthGrades Seventh Annual Patient Safety in American Hospitals Study," March 2010, Appendix C: Patient Safety Incidence Rates and Associated Mortality Among Medicare Beneficiaries (2006-2008).

108. Drew Griffin, telephone interview with the author, 20 April 2011.

109. Kate Suchmann, telephone interview with the author, 20 April 2011.

110. "Bedsores (Pressure Sores) Treatments and Drugs," Mayo Clinic, http://www.mayoclinic.org/diseases-conditions/bedsores/basics/treatment/con-20030848, accessed 29 March 2014.

111. Jill Van Den Bos, Karan Rustagi, Travis Gray, Michael Halford, Eva Ziemkiewicz, and Jonathan Shreve, "The $17.1 Billion Problem: The Annual Cost of Measurable Medical Errors," *Health Affairs*, April 2011, Exhibit 4: "Frequency and Costs of Medicare 'Never Events,' 2008."

112. Kate Suchmann, telephone interview with the author, 20 April 2011.

113. "Hospital-Acquired Conditions (HAC) in Acute Inpatient Prospective Payment System (IPPS) Hospitals," U.S. Department of Health and Human Services, Centers for Medicare & Medicaid Services, October 2012, found at http://www.cms.gov/Medicare/Medicare-Fee-for-Service-Payment/HospitalAcqCond/downloads/HACFactSheet.pdf

114. Robert Galvin, "'A Deficiency of Will and Ambition': A Conversation with Donald Berwick," *Health Affairs*, 12 January 2005.

Chapter 7: "The diagnosis you get is correct"

115. Mark L. Graber, Robert M. Wachter, and Christine K. Cassel, "Bringing Diagnosis Into the Quality and Safety Equations," *JAMA*, 26 September 2012.

116. "Grasping for Straws," *Mystery Diagnosis*, Discovery Health Channel, Season 1, Episode 5, first aired 21 November 2005.

117. Hardeep Singh, Ashley N. D. Meyer, and Eric J. Thomas, "The frequency of diagnostic errors in outpatient care: estimations from three large observational studies involving US adult populations," *BMJ Quality & Safety*, 17 April 2014 (online).

118. Mark L. Graber, Robert M. Wachter, and Christine K. Cassel, "Bringing Diagnosis Into the Quality and Safety Equations," *JAMA*, 26 September 2012.

119. Rosemary Gibson and Janardan Prasad Singh, *Wall of Silence*, Washington, D.C.: Lifeline, 2003.

120. Atul Gawande, *Complications: A Surgeon's Notes on an Imperfect Science*, New York: Henry Holt, 2002. p. 197. "How often do autopsies turn up a major misdiagnosis in the cause of death? . . . According to three studies . . . the figure is about 40 percent. . . . In about a third of the misdiagnoses the patients would have been expected to live if proper treatment had been administered."

See also Lucian L. Leape, "Error in Medicine," *JAMA*, 21 December 1994. "Autopsy studies have shown high rates (35-40 percent) of missed diagnoses causing death."

See also Anahad O'Connor, "Deaths Go Unexamined and the Living Pay the Price," *New York Times*, 02 March 2004. "Autopsies uncover missed or incorrect diagnoses in up to 25 percent of hospital deaths."

See also David Leonhardt, "Why Doctors So Often Get It Wrong," *New York Times*, 22 February 2006. "Studies of autopsies have shown that doctors seriously misdiagnose fatal illnesses about 20 percent of the time. So millions of patients are being treated for the wrong disease."

See also "Diagnostic Error: Is Overconfidence the Problem?" *American Journal of Medicine* Supplement, May 2008. It suggests that diagnostic errors occur 10-15 percent of the time.

See also David E. Newman-Toker and Peter J. Pronovost, "Diagnostic Errors—The Next Frontier for Patient Safety," *JAMA*, 11 March 2009.

121. Owen W. MacDonald, "Physician Perspectives on Preventing Diagnostic Errors," QuantiaMD white paper, September 2011.

122. Atul Gawande, *Complications: A Surgeon's Notes on an Imperfect Science*, New York: Henry Holt, 2002. "How often do autopsies turn up a major misdiagnosis in the cause of death? . . . According to three studies . . . the figure is about 40 percent [of the time] . . .

123. Laura Landro, "What if the Doctor Is Wrong?" *Wall Street Journal*, 17 January 2012.

124. Gary Kantor, "Guest Software Review: Isabel Diagnosis Software," *HIStalk*, 31 January 2006.

See also the website for Isabel Healthcare at www.isabelhealthcare.com/home/default.

125. David Leonhardt, "Why Doctors So Often Get It Wrong," *New York Times*, 22 February 2006.

126. Michael Blastland and Andrew Dilnot, "When Numbers Deceive," *Week*, 27 February 2009, an extract from their book *The Numbers Game*.

127. Ibid.

128. Tara Parker-Pope, "Testing Mistakes at the Family Doctor," *New York Times*, 14 August 2008. The article reports on research published in the journal *Quality & Safety in Health Care*.

129. Questions 3.c. and 3.d. are adapted from a list of three proposed by Jerome Groopman, *How Doctors Think*, Boston: Houghton Mifflin, 2008.

Chapter 8: "You don't need to know what's going on"

130. Vineet Arora, Sandeep Gangireddy, Amit Mehrotra, Ranjan Ginde, Megan Tormey, and David Meltzer, "Ability of Hospitalized Patients to Identify Their In-Hospital Physicians," *Archives of Internal Medicine*, 26 January 2009. Interestingly, 75 percent of patients couldn't name anyone; of the remainder, 60 percent named someone who in fact wasn't involved in their care in the hospital.

131. "The Public Needs to Understand the Uncertainty of Medicines Regulation," *Scrip*, 23 January 2006. These comments were made by Harry Cayton, U.K. Department of

Health Director for Patients and the Public. While he is referring to the U.K., the situation is very similar in the U.S.

132. "'What Did the Doctor Say?' Improving Health Literacy to Protect Patient Safety," Joint Commission, 2007.

133. Daniel R. Beyer, Michael S. Lauer, and Steve Davis, "Letter to the Editor: Readability of Informed-Consent Forms," *New England Journal of Medicine*, 29 May 2003.

134. Kevin J. O'Leary, Nita Kulkarni, Matthew P. Landler, Jiyeon Jeon, Katherine J. Hahn, Katherine M. Englert, and Mark V. Williams, "Hospitalized Patients' Understanding of Their Plan of Care," *Mayo Clinic Proceedings*, February 2010.

135. Laura Landro, "When a Hospital Let Families Call for Rapid-Response Help," *Wall Street Journal*, 31 August 2009.

136. "Problems with Patient Communication Increase Risk for Injury, Death," *Kaiser Daily Health Policy Report*, 26 March 2007. This article describes a news article appearing in *USA Today* that summarizes a report published by the Joint Commission [on Accreditation of Healthcare Organizations], which accredits hospitals.

137. Kevin J. O'Leary, Nita Kulkarni, Matthew P. Landler, Jiyeon Jeon, Katherine J. Hahn, Katherine M. Englert, and Mark V. Williams, "Hospitalized Patients' Understanding of Their Plan of Care," *Mayo Clinic Proceedings*, February 2010.

138. "Health Literacy Overview," Columbia University School of Nursing, http://cumc.columbia.edu/dept/nursing/ebp/HealthLitRes/overview.html, accessed 29 March 2014.

139. Roy P. C. Kesssels, "Patients' Memory for Medical Information," *Journal of the Royal Society of Medicine*, May 2003.

140. Ibid.

141. Ibid.

142. Kevin B. O'Reilly, "The ABCs of Health Literacy," *admednews.com* (American Medical Association), 19 March 2012.

143. Roy P. C. Kesssels, "Patients' Memory for Medical Information," *Journal of the Royal Society of Medicine*, May 2003.

Chapter 9: "Medical records are for doctors"

144. Sharon Sung, "Direct Reporting of Laboratory Test Results to Patients by Mail to Enhance Patient Safety," *Journal of General Internal Medicine*, October 2006. This study revealed that only 14-37 percent of doctors say that they always report normal test results to patients. Only 55-71 percent of doctors say that they always report abnormal results.

See also Tejal K. Gandhi, "Fumbled Handoffs: One Dropped Ball After Another," *Annals of Internal Medicine*, 01 March 2005. Only 25 percent of doctors always tell patients normal results and up to a third don't always tell patients of abnormal results.

145. Melinda Beck, "New Rule Grants Patients Direct Access to Lab Results," *Wall Street Journal*, 03 February 2014.

146. Sharon Sung, "Direct Reporting of Laboratory Test Results to Patients by Mail to Enhance Patient Safety," *Journal of General Internal Medicine*, October 2006.

147. See Chapter 7 for a discussion of false positives. The fact that tests can yield false positives doesn't change the main point. Perhaps 10 people out of 100 will have test results

that suggest that they have cancer. Continuing the example used in Chapter 7, in which 1000 were tested and 99 of 108 people who tested positive did not have the disease, people should be promptly told something like, "About 92% of the people who get a test result like yours don't actually have the disease. On the chance that you might be one of the 8% that does, we need to run another test. Let's do that right away so that the question is settled." The 90 people for whom the test is negative would be relieved to hear this news quickly.

148. Daniel Gilbert, "What You Don't Know Makes You Nervous," *New York Times*, 20 May 2009.

149. Sharon Sung, "Direct Reporting of Laboratory Test Results to Patients by Mail to Enhance Patient Safety," *Journal of General Internal Medicine*, October 2006. This study revealed that only 14-37 percent of doctors say that they always report normal test results to patients. Only 55-71 percent of doctors say that they always report abnormal results.

See also Tejal K. Gandhi, "Fumbled Handoffs: One Dropped Ball After Another," *Annals of Internal Medicine*, 01 March 2005. Only 25 percent of doctors always tell patients normal results and up to a third don't always tell patients of abnormal results.

150. Gina Kolata, "Sick and Scared, and Waiting, Waiting, Waiting," *New York Times*, 20 August 2005. The article goes on to discuss the fact that doctors dismiss as unimportant and not fixable the fact that patients don't like waiting, when solutions are available.

151. Kathleen Fackelmann, "Stress Can Ravage the Body, Unless the Mind Says No," *USA Today*, 22 March 2005.

See also Claudia Dreifus, "Finding Clues to Aging in the Fraying Tips of Chromosomes," *New York Times*, 03 July 2007. Psychological stress causes cells to age, and the aging of the cells is highly correlated with cardiovascular disease and may be correlated with cancer. It appears that stress literally ages people and directly causes many diseases.

152. David H. Freedman, "The Triumph of New-Age Medicine," *Atlantic*, July 2011.

153. Bill Hendrick, "Patients Not Always Told of Lab Results," *WebMD Health News*, 22 June 2009.

154. Lawrence P. Casalino, Daniel Dunham, Marshall H. Chin, Rebecca Bielang, Emily O. Kistner, Theodore G. Karrison, Michael K. Ong, Urmimala Sarkar, Margaret A. McLaughlin, and David O. Meltzer, "Frequency of Failure to Inform Patients of Clinically Significant Outpatient Test Results," *Archives of Internal Medicine*, 22 June 2009. Researchers in one study concluded that doctors fail to report serious abnormal results that call for immediate attention to 7 out of 100 patients. In some academic medical centers, patients were not informed of critical abnormal results in more than 20 percent of the cases.

See also Tejal K. Gandhi, "Fumbled Handoffs: One Dropped Ball After Another," *Annals of Internal Medicine*, 01 March 2005. About a third of patients with abnormal results don't get appropriate follow-up, even if they are told their test results.

See also Traber Davis Giardina and Hardeep Singh, "Should Patients Get Direct Access to Their Laboratory Test Results?" *JAMA*, 14 December 2011.

See also Sharon Sung, "Direct Reporting of Laboratory Test Results to Patients by Mail to Enhance Patient Safety," *Journal of General Internal Medicine*, October 2006.

See also Laura Landro, "U.S. Plan Would Boost Access to Lab Results," *Wall Street Journal*, 20 September 2011.

155. Bill Hendrick, "Patients Not Always Told of Lab Results," *WebMD Health News*, 22 June 2009.

156. Tara Parker-Pope, "Study Equates Stress of Cancer and of Wait for Biopsy Data," *New York Times*, 25 February 2009.

157. "Markle Survey: The Public and Doctors Largely Agree Patients Should Be Able To View, Download and Share Their Health Info," Markle Foundation, January 2011. Despite the optimistic title, only 65 percent of doctors surveyed agreed that "patients should be able to download and keep their own copies of their personal health information." Another 20 percent were neutral and 15 percent disagreed.

158. Paul C. Tang and David Lansky, "The Missing Link: Bridging the Patient-Provider Health Information Gap," *Health Affairs*, September/October 2005.

159. Ibid.

160. Andrea Hassol, James M. Walker, David Kidder, Kim Rokita, David Young, Steven Pierdon, Deborah Deitz, Sarah Kuck, and Eduardo Ortiz, "Patient Experiences and Attitudes about Access to a Patient Electronic Health Care Record and Linked Web Messaging," *Journal of the American Medical Informatics Association*, November/December 2004. "Like paper-based records, EHRs can have problems with accuracy and completeness. In our study, approximately 65 percent of patients rated their personal health information as complete and approximately 75 percent of them rated their medical history as accurate."

161. Pauline W. Chen, "Letting Patients Read the Doctor's Notes," *New York Times*, 04 October 2012.

See also Tom Delbanco, Jan Walker, Sigall K. Bell, Jonathan D. Darer, Joann G. Elmore, Nadine Farag, Henry J. Feldman, Roanne Mejilla, Long Ngo, James D. Ralston, Stephen E. Ross, Neha Trivedi, Elisabeth Vodicka, and Suzanne G. Leveille, "Inviting Patients to Read Their Doctors' Notes: A Quasi-Experimental Study and a Look Ahead" *Annals of Internal Medicine*, 02 October 2012.

See also Laura Landro, "Access to Doctors' Notes Aids Patients' Treatment," *Wall Street Journal*, 01 October 2012.

See also Michael Meltsner, "A Patient's View of OpenNotes," *Annals of Internal Medicine*, 02 October 2012.

See also Kelly Kennedy, "Online access to notes on patients gets mixed reaction," *USA Today*, 19 December 2011.

162. Pauline W. Chen, "Letting Patients Read the Doctor's Notes," *New York Times*, 04 October 2012.

163. Tom Delbanco, Jan Walker, Sigall K. Bell, Jonathan D. Darer, Joann G. Elmore, Nadine Farag, Henry J. Feldman, Roanne Mejilla, Long Ngo, James D. Ralston, Stephen E. Ross, Neha Trivedi, Elisabeth Vodicka, and Suzanne G. Leveille, "Inviting Patients to Read Their Doctors' Notes: A Quasi-Experimental Study and a Look Ahead," *Annals of Internal Medicine*, 02 October 2012.

164. Markle Foundation, "Connecting Americans to Their Health Care," July 2004.

165. "Alternative Diagnosis," http://www.rightdiagnosis.com/intro/overview.htm, downloaded 29 March 2014. "Misdiagnosis can and does occur and is reasonably common with error rates ranging from 1.4 percent in cancer biopsies to a high 20-40 percent misdiagnosis rate in emergency or ICU care."

166. Paul C. Tang and David Lansky, "The Missing Link: Bridging the Patient-Provider Health Information Gap," *Health Affairs*, September/October 2005.

167. Tom Delbanco, Jan Walker, Sigall K. Bell, Jonathan D. Darer, Joann G. Elmore, Nadine Farag, Henry J. Feldman, Roanne Mejilla, Long Ngo, James D. Ralston, Stephen E.

Ross, Neha Trivedi, Elisabeth Vodicka, and Suzanne G. Leveille, "Inviting Patients to Read Their Doctors' Notes: A Quasi-Experimental Study and a Look Ahead" *Annals of Internal Medicine*, 02 October 2012.

168. U.S. Department of Health & Human Services at http://www.hhs.gov/ocr/privacy/hipaa/understanding/consumers/medicalrecords.html. (They point out that the records are available; they don't comment on people's assumptions about that fact.)

169. Victoria E. Knight, "Patient Records Need Reviews," *Wall Street Journal*, 30 August 2007, quoting Joy Pritts, then research associate professor at Georgetown University's Health Policy Institute (no longer providing information about accessing patient records).

Chapter 10: "Doctor knows best"

170. Claudia Dreifus, "Doctor Leads Quest for Safer Ways to Care for Patients," *New York Times*, 08 March 2010.

171. Floyd J. Fowler, Jr., Patricia M. Gallagher, Julie P. W. Bynum, Michael J. Barry, F. Leslie Lucas, and Jonathan S. Skinner, "Decision-Making Process Reported by Medicare Patients Who Had Coronary Artery Stenting or Surgery for Prostate Cancer," *Journal of General Internal Medicine* online, 28 February 2012.

See also a summary by Katherine Hobson, "Surgical Patients Not Getting Information on Alternatives," *Wall Street Journal*, 02 March 2012.

172. Ibid.

173. Peter R. Breggin, *Brain Disabling Treatments in Psychiatry*, New York: Springer, 2008. p. 344.

See also his "Benzodiazepines: Brain-Disabling Effects of Benzodiazepines," on benzo.org.uk, "Adverse reactions to the benzodiazepines as a group: standard textbooks and reviews spanning more than two decades, as well as a variety of clinical studies, confirm widespread recognition of benzodiazepine-induced behavioral abnormalities (DiMascio and Shader, 1970; Kochansky, Salzman, Shader, Harmatz and Ogeltree, 1975; Shader and DiMascio, 1977; Rosenbaum, Woods, Groves et al., 1984; Arana and S. Hyman, 1991; Maxmen, 1991; Maxmen and Ward, 1994; Ashton, 1995)."

174. C. Heather Ashton, "Benzodiazepines: The Still Unfinished Story," speech, 01 November 2000. Ashton is a highly credentialed British doctor and professor.

175. Peter R. Breggin, *Brain Disabling Treatments in Psychiatry*, New York: Springer, 2008. p. 328.

176. David H. Sohn, "Informed Consent: A 'New' Form of Medical Liability?" website of American Academy of Orthopaedic Surgeons/American Association of Orthopaedic Surgeons, accessed 13 March 2014.

177. "Simple, Patient-Friendly Informed Consent Process Increases Proportion of Patients Reading Form and Able to Describe Surgical Procedure," U.S. Department of Health & Human Services, Agency for Healthcare Research and Quality, Innovations Exchange, downloaded 13 March 2014. This study is referring to Melissa M. Bottrell, Hillel Alpert, Ruth L. Fischbach, and Linda L. Emanuel, "Hospital Informed Consent for Procedure: Facilitating Quality Patient-Physician Interaction," *JAMA Surgery (formerly Archives of Surgery)*, January 2000.

178. Floyd J. Fowler, Jr., Patricia M. Gallagher, Julie P. W. Bynum, Michael J. Barry, F.

Leslie Lucas, and Jonathan S. Skinner, "Decision-Making Process Reported by Medicare Patients Who Had Coronary Artery Stenting or Surgery for Prostate Cancer," *Journal of General Internal Medicine* online, 28 February 2012.

179. Rahul K. Parikh, "Showing the Patient the Door, Permanently," *New York Times*, 10 June 2008.

180. Siri Carpenter, "Is Your Parent Over-Medicated?" *Prevention*, December 2008.

181. Michael J. Barry and Susan Edgman-Levitan, "Shared Decision Making—The Pinnacle of Patient-Centered Care," *New England Journal of Medicine*, 01 March 2012.

182. Robert D. Truog, "Patients and Doctors—The Evolution of a Relationship," *New England Journal of Medicine*, 16 February 2012.

183. Michael J. Barry and Susan Edgman-Levitan, "Shared Decision Making—The Pinnacle of Patient-Centered Care," *New England Journal of Medicine*, 01 March 2012. The authors quote Valerie Billingham, a speaker at a seminar called "Through the Patient's Eyes," in 1998.

184. Clarence H. Braddock III, Kelly A. Edwards, Nicole M. Hasenberg, Tracy L. Laidley, and Wendy Levinson, "Informed Decision Making in Outpatient Practice: Time to Get Back to Basics," *JAMA*, 22/29 December 1999.

185. Charles L. Bardes, "Defining 'Patient-Centered Medicine,'" *New England Journal of Medicine*, 01 March 2012.

186. Ibid.

187. A video documenting classroom sessions and their effect on the students can be found at www.pbs.org/wgbh/pages/frontline/shows/divided/.

188. Jared R. Adams, Glyn Elwyn, France Légaré, and Dominick L. Frosch, "Communicating with Physicians about Medical Decisions: A Reluctance to Disagree," *JAMA Internal Medicine* (formerly *Archives of Internal Medicine*), 13/27 August 2012.

189. Dominick L. Frosch, Suepattra G. May, Katharine A. S. Rendle, Caroline Tietbohl, and Glyn Elwyn, "Authoritarian Physicians and Patients' Fear of Being Labeled 'Difficult' Among Key Obstacles To Shared Decision Making," *Health Affairs*, May 2012.

190. Ibid.

191. Laura Landro, "Finding a Way to Ask Doctors Tough Questions," *Wall Street Journal*, 04 March 2009.

192. Dominick L. Frosch, Suepattra G. May, Katharine A. S. Rendle, Caroline Tietbohl, and Glyn Elwyn, "Authoritarian Physicians and Patients' Fear of Being Labeled 'Difficult' Among Key Obstacles To Shared Decision Making," *Health Affairs*, May 2012.

193. Laura Landro, "Finding a Way to Ask Doctors Tough Questions," *Wall Street Journal*, 04 March 2009.

194. Ibid.

195. Jared R. Adams, Glyn Elwyn, France Légaré, and Dominick L. Frosch, "Communicating with Physicians about Medical Decisions: A Reluctance to Disagree," *JAMA Internal Medicine* (formerly *Archives of Internal Medicine*), 13/27 August 2012.

196. Donald F. Phillips, "'New Look' Reflects Changing Style of Patient Safety Enhancement," *JAMA*, 20 January 1999.

197. Clarence H. Braddock III, Kelly A. Edwards, Nicole M. Hasenberg, Tracy L. Laidley, and Wendy Levinson, "Informed Decision Making in Outpatient Practice: Time to Get Back to Basics," *JAMA*, 22/29 December 1999.

198. Marcus C. Korinth, Joachim M. Gilsbach, and Martin R. Weinzierl, "Low-Dose

Aspirin Before Spinal Surgery: Results of a Survey Among Neurosurgeons in Germany," *European Spine Journal*, March 2007. Despite its name, the study reports on data from several European countries.

See also Christopher M. Blanchette, Peter F. Wang, Ashish V. Joshi, Mikael Asmussen, William Saunders, and Peter Kruse, "Cost and Utilization of Blood Transfusions Associated with Spinal Surgeries in the United States," *European Spine Journal*, March 2007.

See also Marc Janssens, Gary Hartstein, and Jean-Louis David, "Reduction in Requirements for Allogenic Blood Products: Pharmacologic Methods," *Annals of Thoracic Surgery*, December 1996. Translated into non-technical terms, the title means that some medicines can reduce bleeding risk and thus reduce the need for blood transfusions.

199. Donald M. Berwick, "Less Is More . . . And Better," *Newsweek*, 16 October 2006. "For many procedures, the variation is stunning. Compared with the lowest-use areas, people in the highest-use areas get 10 times as many prostate operations, six times as many back surgeries, seven times as many coronary angioplasties."

See also John Carey, "Smarter Patients, Cheaper Care?" *Business Week*, 22 June 2009. "'There is good reason to believe 30 percent to 40 percent of what we are spending goes for unnecessary services and inefficient care,' says Dr. Elliott S. Fisher, director of the Center for Health Policy Research at Dartmouth Medical School."

See also Reed Abelson, "Heart Procedure is Off the Charts in an Ohio City," *New York Times*, 18 August 2006.

200. Ibid.

201. Donald M. Berwick, "Less Is More . . . And Better," *Newsweek*, 16 October 2006.

See also "Practice Patterns, Not Patient Needs, Drive Medical Decisions and Cost," *Robert Wood Johnson Foundation Content Alerts*, 27 May 2009.

202. "Supply-Sensitive Care," Dartmouth Atlas Project Topic Brief, http://www.dartmouthatlas.org/topics/supply_sensitive.pdf, accessed 29 March 2014. "Patients . . . in high-spending areas had 82 percent more physician visits, 26 percent more imaging exams, 90 percent more diagnostic tests and 46 percent more minor surgery. Compared to low-intensity regions, patients with hip fractures, colon cancer and heart attacks . . . in high-intensity regions had higher mortality rates and worse 'scorecards' on measures of quality." Most of these studies concern Medicare patients, all insured and with similar coverage.

See also Shannon Brownlee, "Putting Consumers in the Driver's Seat?" AHIP Coverage, 31 May 2005. "In fact, according to a recent study published in the *Annals of Internal Medicine*, mortality in high-cost regions appears to be about two to five percent higher than in the lowest cost regions of the country. The most likely explanation for this is that elderly people who live in high-cost regions spend more time in hospitals than citizens in low-cost regions, and hospitals are risky places, where patients are exposed to the possibility of medical errors, drug interactions, and life-threatening infections."

203. Julie Appleby and Jordan Rau, "Many Hospitals Overuse Double CT Scans, Data Show," *Washington Post*, 18 June 2011.

204. Jane E. Brody, "Medical Radiation Soars, With Risks Often Overlooked," *New York Times*, 20 August 2012.

205. Jane E. Brody, "Medical Radiation Soars, With Risks Often Overlooked," *New York Times*, 20 August 2012.

See also Julie Appleby and Jordan Rau, "Many Hospitals Overuse Double CT Scans, Data Show," *Washington Post*, 18 June 2011.

206. Sandeep Jauhar, "Many Doctors, Many Tests, No Rhyme or Reason," *New York Times*, 11 March 2008.

207. Brian E. Kouri, R. Gregory Parsons, and Hillel R. Alpert, "Physician Self-Referral for Diagnostic Imaging: Review of the Empiric Literature," *American Journal of Roentgenology*, October 2002. "Nonradiologists performing their own imaging are at least 1.7 - 7.7 times as likely to order imaging as non-self-referring physicians in the same specialty who see patients with the same problems."

See also Nicholas Bakalar, "Screening: Doctors Paid for Heart Tests Order More," *New York Times*, 14 November 2011. "A patient of a doctor earning money from testing was more than twice as likely to be tested as a patient of a doctor without financial interest in the tests."

208. Roni Caryn Rabin, "Doctor Panels Recommend Fewer Tests for patients," *New York Times*, 04 April 2012. See earlier notes in this chapter as well.

209. John Carey, "Do Cholesterol Drugs Do Any Good?" *Business Week*, 17 January 2008.

See also Tara Parker-Pope, "A Call for Caution in the Rush to Statins," *New York Times*, 18 November 2008.

See also Jerome Groopman and Pamela Hartzband, "Designing a Smarter Patient," *Wall Street Journal*, 24 September 2011. Without treatment, about 3 out of 100 patients with high cholesterol will have a heart attack over the course of ten years; with treatment with a statin, 2 patients will have heart attacks.

210. John Carey, "Smarter Patients, Cheaper Care?" *Business Week*, 22 June 2009. "'There is good reason to believe 30 percent to 40 percent of what we are spending goes for unnecessary services and inefficient care,' says Dr. Elliott S. Fisher, director of the Center for Health Policy Research at Dartmouth Medical School."

This perspective is routinely echoed by experts around the country.

See also Ceci Connolly, "U.S. 'Not Getting What We Pay For,'" *Washington Post*, 30 November 2008. "As much as half of the $2.3 trillion spent today [on health care in the U.S.] does nothing to improve health." The author quotes a number of health system CEOs and other senior executives, such as the president and CEO of the Mayo Clinic.

See also Brent James, Vice President for Medical Research and Executive Director of the Institute for Healthcare Delivery Research, Intermountain Healthcare, in an address at the 4th Annual World Health Care Congress, 23 April 2007, on "Transformative IT": "32 percent of care provided is inappropriate. Over 50 percent of spending is waste."

See also Peter Lee, President and CEO, Pacific Business Group on Health, in an address at the 4th Annual World Health Care Congress, 23 April 2007 on "Transparency and Public Reporting on the Quality and Cost of Care": "We've seen data that suggests that 50 percent of care is wasted."

See also Julie Appleby, "Consumer Unease with U.S. Health Care Grows," *USA Today*, 16 October 2006. "Overuse and waste can include unnecessary treatments, tests repeated because original results were misplaced or reliance on ineffective treatments. 'Several credible estimates have come up with around 30 percent of health care is unnecessary,' says Richard Deyo, professor of medicine at the University of Washington in Seattle."

See also Gilbert M. Gaul, "Bad Hospitals Net More Money," *Washington Post*, 24 July 2005. "Researchers at Dartmouth Medical School, who have been studying Medicare's performance for three decades, estimate that as much as $1 of every $3 is wasted on unnecessary or inappropriate care. Other analysts put the figure as high as 40 percent."

See also Elliott Fisher, David Goodman, Jonathan Skinner, and Kristen Bronner, "Health Care Spending, Quality, and Outcomes: More Isn't Always Better," Dartmouth Institute for Health Policy & Clinical Practice, A Dartmouth Atlas Project Topic Brief, 27 February 2009.

211. Vinay Prasad, Andrae Vandross, Caitlin Toomey, Michael Cheung, Jason Rho, Steven Quinn, Satish Jacob Chacko, Durga Borkar, Victor Gall, Senthil Selvaraj, Nancy Ho, and Adam Cifu, "A Decade of Reversal: An Analysis of 146 Contradicted Medical Practices," *Mayo Clinic Proceedings*, August 2013.

212. Ibid.

213. Ibid.

Chapter 11: How did we get here?

214. All three licensed images are from www.dollarphotoclub.com. Candlestick phone: image #54137575 Michael Flippo. Mid-20th century phone: image #54825666 olos2013. Smart phone: image #51925170 HuHu Lin. Licensed and downloaded 25 March 2014.

215. "Ten Great Public Health Achievements—United States, 1900-1999," *Morbidity and Mortality Weekly Report*, Centers for Disease Control, 02 April 1999. "During the 20th century, the health and life expectancy of persons residing in the United States improved dramatically. Since 1900, the average lifespan of persons in the United States has lengthened by greater than 30 years; 25 years of this gain are attributable to advances in public health."

See also James W. Henderson, *Health Economics and Policy*, Cincinnati: South-Western, 1999, p. 142. "Research on the relationship between health status and medical care frequently has found that the marginal contribution of medical care to health status is rather small."

See also Sherman Folland, Allen Goodman, and Miron Stano, *The Economics of Health and Health Care*, 3rd ed., Upper Saddle River: Prentice Hall, 2001, p. 118. "The historical declines in population mortality rates were not due to medical interventions because effective medical interventions became available to populations largely after the mortality had declined. Instead, public health, improved environment, and improved nutrition probably played substantial roles."

216. *Health, United States, 2008*, U.S. Department of Health & Human Services, National Center for Health Statistics, 2008. Table 26.

217. Mitchell L. Cohen, "Changing Patterns of Infectious Disease," *Nature*, 17 August 2000. "For most of the twentieth century, the predominant feeling about the treatment, control and prevention of infectious diseases was optimism. In 1931, Henry Sigerist wrote(1), 'Most of the infectious diseases . . . have now yielded up their secrets. . . . Many illnesses . . . had been completely exterminated; others had [been brought] largely under control.' Between 1940 and 1960, the development and successes of antibiotics and immunizations added to this optimism, and in 1969, Surgeon General William H. Stewart(2) told the United States Congress that it was time to 'close the book on infectious diseases.'" [Footnotes within this note can be found in the citation itself.]

218. *Health, United States, 2008*, U.S. Department of Health & Human Services, National Center for Health Statistics, 2008. Table 26.

219. "Chronic Diseases and Health Promotion," Centers for Disease Control and Prevention, http://www.cdc.gov/chronicdisease/overview/index.htm?s_cid=ostltsdyk_ govd_203 accessed 29 March 2014.

220. Ibid.

See also Kathleen Fackelmann, "Stress Can Ravage The Body, Unless The Mind Says No," *USA Today*, 22 March 2005. "Up to 90 percent of the doctor visits in the USA may be triggered by a stress-related illness, says the Centers for Disease Control and Prevention."

See also David H. Freedman, "The Triumph of New-Age Medicine," *Atlantic*, July 2011. The article quotes Elizabeth Blackburn, a Nobel laureate and researcher at the University of California at San Francisco: "Relieving patient stress, in particular, is looking more and more important."

221. *Health, United States, 2012: With Special Feature on Emergency Care*, U.S. Department of Health & Human Services, Centers for Disease Control and Prevention, National Center for Health Statistics. Table 88 (p. 1 of 3). In 2010, 1,008,802,000 office visits are noted.

The U.S. Census Bureau reports at http://quickfacts.census.gov/qfd/states/00000.html, accessed 26 March 2014, a U.S. population in 2010 of about 309,000,000 people, thus an average of about 3.3 visits per person in a year.

222. Sharon Sung, "Direct Reporting of Laboratory Test Results to Patients by Mail to Enhance Patient Safety," *Journal of General Internal Medicine*, October 2006.

223. Ibid.

224. Incidentally, this second solution would also solve the doctors' time problem. Sharon Sung, "Direct Reporting of Laboratory Test Results to Patients by Mail to Enhance Patient Safety," *Journal of General Internal Medicine*, October 2006, also noted that the solutions would differ based on which problem one was attempting to solve: the doctor's time constraint or the failure to report serious abnormal results.

225. The descriptions of process steps related to a doctor's visit and what can go wrong with them are adapted from Elizabeth L. Bewley, "Solving America's Health Care Problems," 1996 (revised, 2010). This white paper is available for free download at http://www. pariohealth.net/Publications.html. Under "Books," select its title.

226. Thomas Bodenheimer, Kate Lorig, Halsted Holman, and Kevin Grumbach, "Patient Self-Management of Chronic Disease in Primary Care," *JAMA*, 20 November 2002. "People with chronic conditions are the principal care-givers. Each day, patients decide what they are going to eat, whether they will exercise and to what extent they will consume prescribed medicines."

227. Jane Brody, "The Importance of Knowing What the Doctor Is Talking About," *New York Times*, 30 January 2007.

228. "Many Americans Disregard Doctors' Course of Treatment," *Wall Street Journal*, 15 March 2007.

229. Laura Landro, "Taking Medical Jargon Out of Doctor Visits," *Wall Street Journal*, 06 July 2010.

230. Noel Gardner, conversation with the author, May 2008. Dr. Gardner has been involved in education of medical students for decades and noted that virtually all students reply with this answer when asked what their job is.

231. *Health, United States, 2012: With Special Feature on Emergency Care*, U.S. Department of Health & Human Services, Centers for Disease Control and Prevention, National Center for Health Statistics. The first two statistics come from Table 88, p. 2 and the third from Table 99.

232. Many people would say that a "customer" is someone who writes the check (so to speak) to buy something. They would conclude that therefore the customer of health care is the government, which pays about half the tab in the United States, and employers, who pay another 25-40 percent, depending on how one counts. For the purpose of this book, customer is defined a bit differently. Health care can change or end people's lives. People have to live in the bodies treated. They also have to take many of the actions required to prevent or treat medical problems. For these reasons, I suggest that they should be viewed as the primary customers of health care.

233. Donald M. Berwick, "What 'Patient-Centered' Should Mean: Confessions of an Extremist," *Health Affairs* online, 19 May 2009.

Chapter 12: When health care is about you

234. David B. Reuben and Mary E. Tinetti, "Goal-Oriented Patient Care—An Alternative Health Outcomes Paradigm," *New England Journal of Medicine*, 01 March 2012.

235. Ibid.

236. Laura Landro, "The Simple Idea That Is Transforming Health Care," *Wall Street Journal*, 16 April 2012.

237. David A. Asch and Kevin G. Volpp, "What Business Are We In? The Emergence of Health as the Business of Health Care," *New England Journal of Medicine*, 29 August 2012.

238. Jacob Goldstein, "MacArthur Genius Award: Reducing Falls in the Elderly," *Wall Street Journal*, 22 September 2009.

See also Karen Pennar, "A Firm Diagnosis of Frailty," *New York Times*, 25 June 2012.

239. Ibid.

240. Mary E. Tinetti, Terri R. Fried, and Cynthia M. Boyd, "Designing Health Care for the Most Common Chronic Condition—Multimorbidity," *New England Journal of Medicine*, 20 June 2012.

241. Siri Carpenter, "Treating an Illness is One Thing. What About a Patient with Many?" *New York Times*, 31 March 2009.

242. Jessica Marcy, "Chronic Disease Expert: U.S. Health Care System Needs To Treat 'Whole Person,'" *Kaiser Health News*, 25 June 2010. Professor Kate Lorig at Stanford University is quoted.

243. American Geriatrics Society Expert Panel on the Care of Older Adults with Multimorbidity, "Guiding Principles for the Care of Older Adults with Multimorbidity," *Journal of the American Geriatrics Society*, Special Articles, 2012.

244. "ED [Emergency Department] Patients More Satisfied If They Know Wait Times," *FierceHealthcare*, 31 July 2008.

245. Nicholas Bakalar, "Reminder to Smokers: Your Lungs Are Aging," *New York Times*, 11 March 2008.

246. Current life expectancy calculators go part of the distance. See, for example, the

Blue Zones Vitality Compass, at http://apps.bluezones.com/vitality/ and Living to 100 at www.livingto100.com. However, they don't factor in treatment choices you make, nor do they add other critical elements: the activities you care about doing and the odds that you'll still be able to do them at various intervals into the future.

247. The second response came from Charles Adler, physician, Mayo Clinic in Arizona, consultation with the author, 03 June 2009.

248. The Mayo Clinic hasn't reached this point by accident. They put a great deal of effort into research to improve the experience of people treated there. See for example Barbara R. Spurrier's presentation in the session, "Signature Innovations to Transform the Delivery and Experience of Health Care," 6th Annual World Health Care Congress, 15 April 2009. Spurrier is Senior Administrator, Center for Innovation, Mayo Clinic.

249. Sharon Begley, "Why Thinking You Got a Workout May Make Your Body Healthier," *Wall Street Journal*, 02 February 2007.

250. Leila Abboud, "Drug Makers Seek to Bar 'Placebo Responders' From Trials," *Wall Street Journal*, 18 June 2004.

251. "Farewell to Scientist Who Discovered Penicillin," BBC, 11 March 1955, found at http://news.bbc.co.uk/onthisday/hi/dates/stories/march/11/newsid_2538000/2538043.stm.

252. "Alexander Fleming," Wikipedia, http://en.wikipedia.org/wiki/Alexander_Fleming, accessed 29 March 2014.

253. "Hawthorne Effect," Wikipedia at http://en.wikipedia.org/wiki/Hawthorne_effect, accessed 30 May 2014.

254. It made news in September 2012 when a major medical school added a department of family medicine. Typically, medical schools have had departments for specialties such as orthopedics and cardiology—but not for primary care. See Jenny Gold, "The Next Frontier for Elite Med Schools: Primary Care," *Kaiser Daily Health Policy Report*, 23 September 2012.

255. Others also note the need to update medical education. See Jacob Goldstein, "What Medical Education Has to Do With Health Reform," *Wall Street Journal*, 16 June 2009. He describes a report published by MedPac, which advises Congress on Medicare: "Specifically, the report cited 'the relative lack of formal training and experience in multidisciplinary teamwork, cost awareness in clinical decision making, comprehensive health information technology, and patient care in ambulatory [non-hospital] settings.' More generally, the report noted, medical residencies are largely based in hospitals." The full report—nearly 300 pages—is titled "Report to the Congress: Improving Incentives in the Medicare Program," at http://www.medpac.gov/documents/Jun09_EntireReport.pdf.

256. American Geriatrics Society Expert Panel on the Care of Older Adults with Multimorbidity, "Guiding Principles for the Care of Older Adults with Multimorbidity: An Approach for Clinicians," *Journal of the American Geriatric Society*, Special Articles, 2012.

See also Siri Carpenter, "Treating an Illness is One Thing. What About a Patient with Many?" *New York Times*, 31 March 2009.

See also Siri Carpenter, "Is Your Parent Over-Medicated?" *Prevention*, December 2008.

257. American Geriatrics Society Expert Panel on the Care of Older Adults with Multimorbidity, "Guiding Principles for the Care of Older Adults with Multimorbidity: An Approach for Clinicians," *Journal of the American Geriatric Society*, Special Articles, 2012.

See also www.healthinaging.org.

See also Rosanne M. Leipzig, "The Patients Doctors Don't Know," *New York Times*, 02 July 2009.

258.   Dennis McCullough, *My Mother, Your Mother: Embracing "Slow Medicine," the Compassionate Approach to Caring for Your Aging Loved One*, New York: Harper, 2008.

259.   Clarence H. Braddock III, Kelly A. Edwards, Nicole M. Hasenberg, Tracy L. Laidley, and Wendy Levinson, "Informed Decision Making in Outpatient Practice: Time to Get Back to Basics," *JAMA*, 22-29 December 1999.

260.   Laura Landro, "Weighty Choices, in Patients' Hands," *Wall Street Journal*, 04 August 2009.

See also John Carey, "Smarter Patients, Cheaper Care?" *Business Week*, 22 June 2009. The article is subtitled, "Better-informed medical decisions could cut billions in health-care costs as patients opt for cheaper treatments."

261.   Richard M. Hoffman, Mick P. Couper, Brian J. Zikmund-Fisher, Carrie A. Levin, Mary McNaughton-Collins, Deborah L. Helitzer, John VanHoewyk, and Michael J. Barry, "Prostate Cancer Screening Decisions," *Archives of Internal Medicine*, 28 September 2009. In this case, "Health care providers emphasized the pros of testing in 71.4 percent of discussions but infrequently addressed the cons (32.0 percent)." This kind of disparity is common across testing and treatment discussions for many conditions.

262.   Michael K. Paasche-Orlow, Holly A. Taylor, and Frederick L. Brancati, "Readability Standards for Informed-Consent Forms as Compared with Actual Readability," *New England Journal of Medicine*, 20 February 2003, notes, "Almost half of Americans read at or below the 8th-grade level." The article goes on to suggest the use of materials written at a 4th-grade level.

See also Nancy Cotugna, Connie E. Vickery, and Kara M. Carpenter-Haefele, "Evaluation of Literacy Level of Patient Education Pages in Health-Related Journals," *Journal of Community Health*, June 2005.

See also "'What Did the Doctor Say?': Improving Health Literacy to Protect Patient Safety," Joint Commission, 2007.

See also Mark Kutner, Elizabeth Greenberg, Ying Jin, and Christine Paulsen, "The Health Literacy of America's Adults: Results from the 2003 National Assessment of Adult Literacy," project officer Sheida White, National Center for Education Statistics, U.S. Department of Education, September 2006.

Chapter 13: What will it take to fix health care?

263.   This note calculates the number of deaths due to health care each year in the United States, including those from hospital-related infections, blood clots, and medical errors and from adverse drug events both in and out of the hospital. Discussion follows the details.

Infections Due To Hospital Care
"Data and Statistics: HAI Prevalence Survey," Centers for Disease Control and Prevention, http://www.cdc.gov/HAI/surveillance/, quoting a *New England Journal of Medicine* study, "Multistate Point-Prevalence Survey of Health Care-Associated Infections," published 27

March 2014, which concluded that about 722,000 people pick up infections in hospitals every year, and 75,000 of them die as a direct result.

Blood Clots Due To Hospital Care
John A. Heit, Alexander T. Cohen, and Frederick A. Anderson, Jr., on behalf of the VTE Impact Assessment Group, "Estimated Annual Number of Incident and Recurrent, Non-Fatal and Fatal Venous Thromboembolism (VTE) Events in the US," *Blood* 2005 (American Society of Hematology (ASH) Annual Meeting Abstracts) Abstract #910.

This document reports 189,819 total fatalities annually from deep vein thrombosis and pulmonary embolisms related to hospital care, so 190K is used in the text.

See also Laura Landro, "In the Hospital, Facing a Scourge of Killer Clots," *Wall Street Journal*, 01 April 2009: "Deep-vein thrombosis followed by pulmonary embolism . . . kills nearly 200,000 U.S. patients a year."

Heit and fellow researchers provided the following annualized counts of blood clots of two types (pulmonary embolism or PE and deep vein thrombosis or DVT), separated into fatal and non-fatal instances and whether they arose from hospitalization or not:

Blood clots in the U.S.

Type	Hospital	Community	Total
Non-Fatal DVT	268,125	108,240	376,365
Non-Fatal PE	151,700	85,358	237,058
Total Non-Fatal	**419,825**	**193,598**	**613,423**
Fatal DVT	1,609	649	2,258
Fatal PE	188,210	105,902	294,112
Total Fatal	**189,819**	**106,551**	**296,370**
Grand Total	**609,644**	**300,149**	**909,793**

Medical Errors in Hospitals
"HealthGrades Quality Study Patient Safety in American Hospitals 2004," reports, "excluding obstetric patients, we calculated that over 575,000 preventable deaths occurred . . . in U.S. hospitals from 2000 through 2002."

Please note three points: first, this calculation excludes obstetrics. Second, these are problems from *preventable* deaths from medical errors; most of the other calculations do not distinguish between preventable and non-preventable deaths, so these numbers are lower than they would be if they were consistent in structure with the rest of the numbers used. Third, there is overlap with infections and blood clots here; these double counts are subtracted out later, below.

The HealthGrades study identifies deaths due to the following problems: accidental puncture or laceration, complications of anesthesia, death in low mortality Diagnostic Related Grouping (DRGs), decubitus ulcer (bedsores), failure to rescue, foreign body left during procedure, iatrogenic pneumothorax (collapsed lung), selected infections due to medical care, transfusion reaction, and these post-operative complications: hemorrhage or hematoma, hip fracture, physiologic and metabolic derangement, pulmonary embolism or deep vein thrombosis (blood clots), respiratory failure, sepsis, and wound dehiscence.

See also Laura Landro, "Report Card to Rank Hospitals on Safety," *Wall Street Journal*, 22 April 2004: "The incidence of medical errors is higher than some patients might think. The Institute of Medicine reported in 2000 that medical errors cause as many as 98,000 deaths annually, but some safety experts now say the report actually understates the problem. . . . A more realistic number may be as high as 200,000 deaths per year.'"

Paul Davies, "Fatal Medical Errors Said To Be More Widespread," *Wall Street Journal*, 27 July 2004: "A new study coming out today . . . estimated that medical errors in U.S. hospitals contributed to almost 600,000 patient deaths over the past three years, double the number of deaths from a study published in 2000 by the Institute of Medicine."

Based on the above, 200K is used in the text.

Medication Side Effects

Three studies are highlighted below.

Saul Weingart, Ross McL. Wilson, Robert W. Gibberd, and Bernadette Harrison, "Epidemiology of Medical Error," *BMJ*, 18 March 2000: Adverse drug events among people not in hospitals "accounted for . . . 199,000 additional deaths."

Frank R. Ernst and Amy J. Grizzle, "Drug-Related Morbidity and Mortality: Updating the Cost-of-Illness Model," *Journal of the American Pharmaceutical Association*, March/April 2001, reports that side effects of drugs in people not in hospitals accounted for 218,113 deaths.

Both of these studies also reported other consequences of side effects, listed below.

Side effects of medicines in patients who are not hospitalized

Result of drug side effects	Weingart	Ernst	Average
Physician visits	116,000,000	126,846,567	**121,423,284**
Additional prescriptions	76,000,000	83,735,556	**79,867,778**
Emergency dept visits	17,000,000	18,703,833	**17,851,917**
Hospital admissions	8,000,000	9,609,722	**8,804,661**
Long-term care admissions	3,000,000	3,454,460	**3,227,230**
Deaths	199,000	218,113	**208,557**

Jason Lazarou, Bruce Pomeranz, and Paul N. Corey, "Incidence of Adverse Drug Reactions in Hospitalized Patients: A Meta-Analysis of Prospective Studies," *JAMA*, 15 April, 1998: "We estimate that in 1994, . . . 106,000 . . . [hospitalized patients] had fatal ADRs [adverse drug reactions] making these reactions between the fourth and sixth leading cause of death." They note that the 106,000 reflects a range of 76,000-137,000. This study defines an adverse drug reaction more narrowly than other studies define adverse drug events.

Taking together the average of the deaths due to drug side effects in non-hospitalized patients from the chart above and Lazarou's numbers for hospitalized patients yields:

Deaths due to side effects of medicines

Non-Hospitalized (average)	Hospitalized	Total
208,557	106,000	**314,557**

Discussion

One must subtract possible double counts in the medical error numbers. To do so, I used the deaths for Medicare patients attributable to infections and blood clots included in the HealthGrades medical error numbers—HealthGrades being the only one of the studies that offered this level of detail—and, using the HealthGrades estimate that 45 percent of the relevant hospital population is on Medicare, grossed these deaths up to estimate the numbers for the total population that may be double counted as follows:

Possible double counts

Blood clots	19,000
Infections	8,000
Sepsis	11,000
Total possible double counts	38,000

I included the sepsis number to be safe, although it may not in fact be a double count. Using the lower number for non-hospitalized patient deaths due to drug side effects, and subtracting possible double counts, at a minimum the numbers are:

Total deaths due to selected health care causes

Type	Number/Year
Medical errors in hospitals	200,000
Blood clots in hospitals	190,000
Infections in hospitals	75,000
Drug side effects in hospitals	106,000
Drug side effects not in hospitals	199,000
Subtotal—selected causes	**770,000**
Less possible double counts	(38,000)
Net total—selected causes	**732,000**

Compare these numbers to the leading diseases listed as causes of death nationally:

Top four diseases causing death

Heart disease	596,000
Cancer	575,000
Chronic lower respiratory diseases	143,000
Stroke	129,000

The data on deaths (rounded) comes from Donna L. Hoyert and Jiaquan Xu, "Deaths: Preliminary Data for 2011," National Vital Statistics Reports, 10 October 2012, found at http://www.cdc.gov/nchs/data/nvsr/nvsr61/nvsr61_06.pdf.

Note that the number of 732,000 deaths calculated above due to side effects and complications of health care means that health care is the leading cause of death in America, by a wide margin. According to the same federal government report noted above, about 2.513 million people die each year in America. Thus, 29 percent of all deaths in this country appear to be caused by medical care.

Of course, everyone dies of something—eventually—but in many cases, deaths resulting from health care come years or even decades before the individuals would be expected to die were it not for side effects and complications.

Exclusions from the Count of Deaths Due to Health Care

Except for drug side effects, the figures above are hospital-based. Little research has been done on the harm that health care causes outside of the hospital. However, consider Tara F. Bishop, Andrew M. Ryan, and Lawrence P. Casalino, "Paid Malpractice Claims for Adverse Events in Inpatient and Outpatient Settings," JAMA, 15 June 2011. They observed that roughly equal numbers of malpractice claims were paid for inpatients and for outpatients in the U.S. in the five years ending in 2009. The authors suggest that health care may result in as much harm outside of hospital settings as inside.

About 12 million people suffer adverse events in the hospital, derived as follows: the Institute for Healthcare Improvement concluded that about a third of the time when people were in the hospital, they experienced at least one adverse event. See Donald M. Berwick, plenary presentation "Mont Sainte-Victoire" at the Institute for Healthcare Improvement 18th Annual National Forum on Quality Improvement in Health Care, Orlando, FL, 12 December 2006.

Counting only the 37 million inpatient stays (that is, ignoring the 130 million emergency room visits and the 101 million hospital outpatient visits), the above means that over 12 million people a year suffer an adverse event in the hospital.

If an equal number, or 12 million, are harmed outside hospitals, one might then want to know how many of them die. If the patterns revealed in the Institute for Healthcare Improvement research apply outside the hospital, about 11% of these events might cause permanent harm (including death). But research is not available to confirm this very rough estimate that is suggested here simply to help frame the discussion.

Consider also Tara Parker-Pope, "Testing Mistakes at the Family Doctor," New York Times, 14 August 2008. The article mentions in passing that "medical errors or adverse events in family practices occur in about one in four patient visits," but does not identify the studies that led to that conclusion or indicate how serious the errors are.

As noted in Chapter 7, one recently published study estimated deaths due to misdiagnosis as roughly 40,000 to 80,000 people per year. See Mark L. Graber, Robert M. Wachter, and Christine K. Cassel, "Bringing Diagnosis Into the Quality and Safety Equations," JAMA, 26 September 2012.

According to Dr. Wes Ely, a leading researcher in the field of hospital-related delirium, in the first six months after discharge, people who developed delirium in the hospital die at three times the rate of a matched cohort whose members did not develop delirium in the hospital. See E. Wesley Ely, "ICU Delirium Epidemiology, Monitoring, & Manage-

ment," slide presentation, 2006. http://www.mc.vanderbilt.edu/icudelirium/docs/ICU_
slides_02_2006.pdf.

Deaths that result directly from mistakes such as misdiagnosis or hospital-acquired delirium may occur weeks or months after the episode of care in which the mistake or error in care took place. These deaths are not included above in the calculations of deaths caused by health care.

The list goes on. For example, infections or medical errors that kill people at other sites such as nursing homes are not included in the counts.

Despite these obvious omissions, I have not added estimates for deaths caused by side effects and complications outside of hospitals, except for the adverse drug events specifically listed separately above. The numbers that are included should be sufficient to make the point: a very large number of people are injured or killed by the care they receive.

264. According to the U.S. Census Bureau, http://quickfacts.census.gov/qfd/states/25/2507000.html and http://quickfacts.census.gov/qfd/states/25/2511000.html, accessed 29 March 2014, population estimates for 2012 for the Massachusetts cities of Boston and Cambridge are 636,479 and 106,471, respectively. These total 742,950, roughly equivalent to the 732,000 listed for deaths from selected causes of health care.

265. The statistic comes from a patient education brochure prepared by the ICU Delirium and Cognitive Impairment Study Group, run by Dr. Wes Ely of Vanderbilt University Medical Center and found at http://www.mc.vanderbilt.edu/icudelirium/docs/delirium_education_brochure.pdf, accessed 29 March 2014. While "insane" is not a clinical term, it is defined by one dictionary as "in a state of mind that prevents normal perception, behavior, or social interaction," which delirium, the topic here, certainly does.

Appendix A: Why won't the usual solutions work?

266. Versions of this story appear at http://www.geocities.com/Tokyo/Courtyard/1652/Elephant.html and http://www.milk.com/random-humor/elephant_fable.html. The version in *When Health Care Hurts* is an amalgam of the two.

267. Consider the perspective in "Health Care's Infectious Losses," by Paul O'Neill, *New York Times*, 06 July 2009: "Which of the [health reform] proposals will eliminate the annual toll of 300 million medication errors? . . . Which of the proposals will capture even a fraction of the roughly $1 trillion of annual 'waste' that is associated with the kinds of process failures [questions like this] imply? So far, the answer . . . is 'none.'"

Additionally, there is limited research to indicate that many of these solutions actually move the dial.

For example, see Sumit R. Majumdar and Stephen B. Soumerai, "The Unhealthy State of Health Policy Research," *Health Affairs* online, 11 August 2009. This article describes the flawed research that creates unsupported claims that Health Information Technology, Pay for Performance, and increased cost-sharing (Consumer-Directed Health Plans) yield improved results.

See also "Study Questions Effectiveness of Pay-for-Performance System," *Kaiser Daily Health Policy Report*, 10 March 2009.

See also Steffie Woolhandler and Dan Ariely, "Will Pay for Performance Backfire? Insights from Behavioral Economics," *Health Affairs* blog, 11 October 2012. "Researchers have been unable to show that [Pay for Performance] benefits patients."

268. Arnold Milstein, "Toxic Waste in the U.S. Health System," *Health Affairs* blog, 02 June 2008. Milstein notes that 24,000 people a year were expected to die as a result of lack of insurance. Contrast this number with the 732,000 deaths from medical errors, hospital-acquired infections, and other care-related problems summarized in Chapter 13. About six times as many people have insurance as don't have insurance, so these numbers mean that if the people without coverage became insured, and quality of care stayed about the same, then about another 122,000 people a year would die due to complications of care, far exceeding the 24,000 who die today because they don't have insurance.

That's not an argument for keeping people uninsured; it does suggest, however, that the primary issues with quality of care are not financial.

See also Elizabeth Docteur and Robert A. Berenson, "How Does the Quality of U.S. Health Care Compare Internationally?" Robert Wood Johnson Foundation, August 2009, which notes, "If reform accomplishes no more than extending insurance coverage to the more than 45 million Americans without insurance, it will be an important step forward, but more is needed to ensure health care quality improvement."

269. Uwe Reinhardt, "Why Does U.S. Health Care Cost So Much? (Part II: Indefensible Administrative Costs)," *New York Times*, 21 November 2008. The article quotes a study by McKinsey from 2003, which Reinhardt extrapolates to 2008, estimating that unnecessary spending on administration was $150 billion in 2008. McKinsey estimated that 85 percent of the excess spending on administration is related to the private insurance system. Thus, $150 billion x .85 = roughly $128 billion. Other researchers come up with even bigger numbers, but this one is big enough to make the point.

270. The math is drawn from "In Amenable Mortality—Deaths Avoidable Through Health Care—Progress In The US Lags That Of Three European Countries," by Ellen Nolte and C. Martin McKee, *Health Affairs*, September 2012. In France, 60.97 men and 49.39 women out of every 1,000 age 74 and younger die of conditions that could have been prevented/treated to forestall death. In the U.S., 106.9 men and 84.5 women die. Thus in France these deaths total about 110/2 = 55 per 1,000 and in the U.S. they total about 191/2 = 96 per 1,000. Thus one might say that there are 96/55 = 175 percent = 75 percent more deaths in the U.S. than in France that could have been prevented with appropriate care.

271. Gardiner Harris, "Prosecutors Plan Crackdown on Doctors Who Accept Kickbacks," *New York Times*, 04 March 2009.

272. Robert Pear, "Obama Push to Cut Health Costs Faces Tough Odds," *New York Times*, 12 May 2009. "Such cost-control devices have proved spectacularly ineffective in limiting the growth of Medicare spending on doctors' services."

273. "Birth Control Prices Soar on Campus," *MSNBC*, 23 March 2007.

274. "Decrease Price . . . Increase Supply?" *Healthcare Economist*, 27 October 2006. "When Medicare decides to reduce its fees, the quantity of medical services supplied by physicians actually increases."

275. See Chapter 9.

276. Andrew Pollack, "The Minimal Impact of a Big Hypertension Study," *New York Times*, 28 November 2008.

See also David Pittman, "Effectiveness Research Slow to Change Practice," *MedPage Today*, 09 October 2012, for similar results for some coronary care and knee surgery.

277. Tara Parker-Pope, "A Hurdle for Health Reform: Patients and Their Doctors," *New York Times*, 03 March 2009.

See also Gardiner Harris, "Document Details Plan to Promote Costly Drug," *New York Times*, 02 September 2009, which starts off, "The pharmaceutical industry has developed thousands of medicines that have saved millions of lives, but it has also used its marketing muscle to successfully peddle expensive pills that are no more effective than older drugs sold at a fraction of the cost."

278. "Fewer Patients Using Health Care Provider Quality Ratings Web Sites to Make Decisions," *Kaiser Daily Health Policy Report*, 02 December 2008.

See also "2008 Update on Consumers' Views of Patient Safety and Quality Information," Kaiser Family Foundation, October 2008, which notes, "The share of the public now saying that they have seen and/or used information comparing the quality among various health care related providers has fallen back to levels last recorded in 2000."

279. "Health Care Costs: A Primer—Key Information on Health Care Costs and Their Impact," Kaiser Family Foundation, May 2012.

280. Atul Gawande, "The Cost Conundrum," *New Yorker*, 01 June 2009, quoting a cardiac surgeon.

281. For a discussion of traditional quality measures in health care, see Anthony R. Kovner, *Health Care Delivery in the United States*, 4th ed., New York: Springer, 1990.

282. Steffie Woolhandler and Dan Ariely, "Will Pay for Performance Backfire? Insights from Behavioral Economics," *Health Affairs* blog, 11 October 2012. "Researchers have been unable to show that [Pay for Performance] benefits patients."

283. Regina Herzlinger, *Market-Driven Health Care: Who Wins, Who Loses in the Transformation of America's Largest Service Industry*, New York: Addison-Wesley, 1997.

284. Michael E. Porter and Elizabeth Olmsted Teisberg, *Redefining Health Care: Creating Value-Based Competition on Results*, Boston: Harvard Business School, 2006.

285. Siri Carpenter, "Treating an Illness Is One Thing. What About a Patient With Many?" *New York Times*, 31 March 2009. It notes that 68 percent of dollars spent by Medicare pay for care for "people who have five or more chronic diseases."

286. "PCMH Standards and Guidelines 2014," National Committee for Quality Assurance (NCQA) Patient-Centered Medical Home (PCMH) 2014 Standards, 24 March 2014.

287. Carlos Roberto Jaén, Robert L. Ferrer, William L. Miller, Raymond F. Palmer, Robert Wood, Marivel Davila, Elizabeth E. Stewart, Benjamin F. Crabtree, Paul A. Nutting, and Kurt C. Stange, "Patient Outcomes at 26 Months in the Patient-Centered Medical Home National Demonstration Project," *Annals of Family Medicine*, vol. 8, Supplement 1, September 2010. "There were no significant improvements in patient-rated outcomes, including ratings of the 4 pillars of primary care (easy access to first-contact care, comprehensive care, coordination of care, and personal relationship over time), global practice experience, patient empowerment, and self-rated health status. There were trends for very small decreases in coordination of care, . . . comprehensive care, . . . and access to first-contact care."

288.   Pauline W. Chen, "Putting Patients at the Center of the Medical Home," *New York Times*, 15 July 2010.

Appendix B: An aside on the role of the patient

289. Chris Browne, "Hagar the Horrible," *Daily Courier*, 27 February 2009.

290. Roni Caryn Rabin, "Bad Habits Asserting Themselves," *New York Times*, 09 June 2009. Consider the percentages of people age 40-74 who engage in these healthy behaviors:

Eat five fruits and vegetables a day	26%
Don't smoke	84%
Exercise 30 minutes 3x a week	43%

Multiplying these together yields the conclusion that 9.4 percent did all three.

Then, from "Health Behaviors of Adults: United States 2002-2004," U.S. Department of Health & Human Services, Centers for Disease Control and Prevention, National Center for Health Statistics, Vital and Health Statistics, Series 10, Number 230, September 2006, it develops that 61 percent of the population drinks (Table 3.1) and 20 percent of them have had more than five drinks in a single day in the last year (Table 3.3.) This means that, understating the case somewhat, .61 x .20 = 12 percent of the population might be considered problem drinkers, yielding 88 percent who are not. Factoring this in to the calculation above, about 8 percent of the population is doing well on all four measures.

Statisticians may object that the behaviors listed above may not be independent variables—that is, perhaps people who don't smoke also tend to eat more vegetables. Despite this possibility, the general picture remains.

See also Dana E. King, Arch G. Mainous III, Mark Carnemolla, and Charles J. Everett, "Adherence to Healthy Lifestyle Habits in US Adults, 1988-2006," *American Journal of Medicine*, June 2009. It paints a bleaker picture: "Only 3 percent of US adults adhered to 4 healthy lifestyle characteristics (5 fruits and vegetables a day, regular physical activity, maintaining a healthy weight, and not smoking)."

291. Ron French, "Losing the Battle of the Bulge," *Detroit News*, 27 September 2006.

292. Assume 37 million hospital stays averaging 6 days each, per *Health, United States, 2008*, U.S. Department of Health & Human Services, Centers for Disease Control and Prevention, National Center for Health Statistics, 2008, Table 106. Further assume that each individual is visited 20 times a day by various care providers. That's 37,000,000 stays x 6 days x 20 interactions with care providers = 4,440,000,000 opportunities to pick up an infection. (That's 4.4 billion.)

According to the CDC, 722,000 people pick up infections in the hospital each year and 75,000 die. See "Data and Statistics: HAI Prevalence Survey," Centers for Disease Control and Prevention, http://www.cdc.gov/HAI/surveillance/, quoting a *New England Journal of Medicine* study, "Multistate Point-Prevalence Survey of Health Care-Associated Infections," published 27 March 2014.

One simplified way to look at the numbers is this: 722,000 of the 4,440,000,000 contacts resulted in transmission of a perceptible infection. That's 1 out of every 6,150 contacts. And it means that infections that cause deaths are passed on to patients 75,000 times out of 4.4 billion encounters. That's one out of every 59,000 times.

The number of daily contacts is probably understated by a significant number. Just delivering and picking up meal trays requires six contacts a day. If the number of contacts is larger, then the percentages of contacts that result in infections and deaths from infection is smaller than calculated here. The point remains that people get infections from care providers much less often than they themselves fail to take basic steps to preserve their own health.

293. "Wash Your Hands. No, *Really.*" *Prevention*, March 2009.

294. *Health, United States, 2008*, U.S. Department of Health & Human Services, Centers for Disease Control and Prevention, National Center for Health Statistics, 2008. Table 108 notes that "all employed civilians" in 2007 total 146,047,000. Health care employment for 2007 was 14,687,000 people.

See also Gerald F. Seib, "U.S. Psyche Bedevils Health Effort," *Wall Street Journal*, 04 August 2009, which notes that not only are there more than 14 million jobs in health care today, but the health care industry is expected to add "a staggering three million new wage and salaried jobs in the next decade or so, more than any other industry."

295. "National Health Expenditures 2012 Highlights" found at http://www.cms.gov/ Research-Statistics-Data-and-Systems/Statistics-Trends-and-Reports/NationalHealthExpendData/downloads/highlights.pdf reports, "In 2012 U.S. health care spending increased 3.7 percent to reach $2.8 trillion, or $8,915 per person, the fourth consecutive year of slow growth. The share of the economy devoted to health spending decreased from 17.3 percent in 2011 to 17.2 percent in 2012, as the Gross Domestic Product increased nearly one percentage point faster than health care spending at 4.6 percent."

296. "National Health Expenditures 2012 Highlights" found at http://www.cms.gov/ Research-Statistics-Data-and-Systems/Statistics-Trends-and-Reports/NationalHealthExpendData/downloads/highlights.pdf.

297. Paul Otellini, "Making Health Care Personal," *Politico*, 27 July 2009. The author is CEO of Intel Corp.

298. Statisticians among you may argue that in this hypothetically better world, there would be a big dip in the number of deaths caused by health care that would last for some years, but that eventually the numbers would rise again as people who didn't die from complications of care at, say, age 50 instead died of old age at, say, age 85, engaging the health care system intensively in the last year of life as is often the case today (if nothing else changed in the meantime) and at that point being subjected to the same probability of harm as the 50-year-old is today.

Index

The five indexes, which start on the following page, highlight:

"How To" Action Guides
Sad But True statistics
Figures
Stories
General content

Topic	Sad But True	Page
Bedsores	45,046 deaths in hospitalized Medicare patients in 3 years	66
Bedsores	100% preventable	67
Blood clots	190,000 people die of hospital-related blood clots each year	12
Delirium	60% of 40-60 year olds become delirious in the hospital	20
Delirium	66-84% undiagnosed	21
Delirium	30 seconds is all it takes to diagnose	22
Delirium	10 years of permanent mental decline likely afterwards	23
Delirium	Can be reduced 50% with earplugs	24
Disagreement	15% of patients think disagreeing can yield good outcomes	127
Disrespect	Evidence abounds of demeaning behavior by physicians	60
Disrespect	1 in 9 doctors say they see other doctors behave this way daily	61
Disrespect	26% of doctors admit to behaving this way themselves	62
Disrespect	#1 reason health care fails to reduce harm it causes patients	63
Drugs	1 drug error per day on average for hospital patients	5
Drugs	89% of patients are not warned about side effects	36
Drugs	1 of 4 patients experience side effects within 3 months	37
Drugs	50 common drugs are known to cause weight gain	38
Drugs	Patients may gain up to 100 pounds as a drug side effect	39
Drugs	80% of the time, doctors missed known side effects	40
Drugs	17-19 million people/year land in the ER due to side effects	41
Drugs	Doctors reported only 10% of side effects	42
Drugs	6% of people were helped by antibiotics for sinusitis, 12% hurt	50
Drugs	90% of drugs work in only 30-50% of people taking them	52
Excess	40% of people who got pacemakers got no benefit	51
Excess	65% of hip implants are put in people likely to be harmed	54
Excess	29% of hip implants had to be removed within 6 years	55
Excess	6x-10x increased chance of surgery based on city	131
Excess	2x-8x more tests ordered when doctors own testing service	132
Excess	30-50% of all tests and treatments might be wasted	133
Hospitals	1 in 7 patients age 65+ harmed or killed by hospital care	2
Hospitals	1 in 3 hospital admissions result in harm to patients	3
Hospitals	98% of time, hospitals did not fix problems that hurt patients	17
Hospitals	34% of Medicare patients are readmitted within 30 days	31
Infections	35% of care workers wash hands before touching patients	7

Topic	Sad But True	Page
Infections	75,000 people die of infections they pick up in the hospital	9
Med. Records	14-37% of normal test results are released to patients	98
Med. Records	55-71% of abnormal test results are released to patients	99
Med. Records	0-26% (avg 7%) badly abnormal results don't get to patients	100
Med. Records	Stress is equal for people diagnosed with cancer and people waiting for their cancer test results	101
Med. Records	65% of doctors agree people should be able to get records	102
Med. Records	1 in 4 people found errors in their medical records	103
Med. Records	94% of patients think they should have online records access	104
Med. Records	Up to 80% of docs are "frightened" by this possibility	105
Med. Records	Patients have legal right to records but may not know it	106
Misdiagnosis	10-20% of diagnoses are wrong, missed, or late	74
Misdiagnosis	12 million outpatients misdiagnosed annually, half the time with the potential for severe harm	75
Misdiagnosis	40,000-80,000 people die yearly due to wrong diagnoses	76
Misdiagnosis	1 in 3 people found in autopsies to be misdiagnosed would probably have lived if diagnosed correctly and treated	77
Misdiagnosis	96% of doctors say misdiagnosis could often be prevented	78
Misdiagnosis	75+ years that rates of misdiagnosis have stayed the same	79
Misdiagnosis	100+ physical conditions can appear to be psychological	80
Misdiagnosis	92% of doctors badly misinterpreted accuracy of test results	81
Process	54% chance that a process with 12 steps will be done right	144
Ranks	Health care reported as 3rd leading cause of death (but study omitted some causes such as blood clots and misdiagnosis)	6
Ranks	U.S. ranked last (19th out of 19 countries) in preventing preventable deaths	10
Ranks	U.S. ranks 42nd in the world in life expectancy	13
Recall	14% of information given orally is recalled by patients	92
Recall	40-80% of what doctors say is typically forgotten right away	93
Recall	Half of the information patients remember is incorrect	96
Uninformed	90% of hospital patients didn't know who was in charge of their care	86
Uninformed	55% of patients believed they had diagnoses that they didn't	87
Uninformed	48% of hospital patients thought they were getting tests different from what the doctor actually ordered	88
Uninformed	41-75% did not understand informed consent forms	90

(Family members' names appear in parentheses when they provided the narratives.)